Routledge Revivals

The Elements of Vital Statistics

First published in 1889, this book provides a guide to vital statistics- the science of numbers applied to the life-history of communities and nations- in relation to medical problems. Chapters cover a wide variety of categories including population, births and deaths, sickness, occupation and mortality, and mortality from special diseases.

The Elements of Vital Statistics

Sir Arthur Newsholme

Routledge Revivals
Routledge
Taylor & Francis Group

First published in 1889
by Swan Sonnenschein & Co.

This edition first published in 2015 by Routledge
2 Park Square, Milton Park, Abingdon, Oxon, OX14 4RN
and by Routledge
711 Third Avenue, New York, NY 10017

Routledge is an imprint of the Taylor & Francis Group, an informa business

Publisher's Note
The publisher has gone to great lengths to ensure the quality of this reprint but points out that some imperfections in the original copies may be apparent.

Disclaimer
The publisher has made every effort to trace copyright holders and welcomes correspondence from those they have been unable to contact.

A Library of Congress record exists under LC control number: 05021124

ISBN 13: 978-1-138-90656-3 (hbk)
ISBN 13: 978-1-315-69541-9 (ebk)
ISBN 13: 978-1-138-90658-7 (pbk)

THE ELEMENTS

OF

VITAL STATISTICS

BY

ARTHUR NEWSHOLME, M.D., LOND.,

UNIVERSITY SCHOLAR IN MEDICINE; CERTIF. IN PUBLIC HEALTH UNIV. LOND.;
FELLOW OF THE ROYAL STATISTICAL SOCIETY;
MEDICAL OFFICER OF HEALTH FOR BRIGHTON; LATE MEDICAL OFFICER
OF HEALTH FOR CLAPHAM; AUTHOR OF MANUALS OF
"HYGIENE," AND OF "SCHOOL HYGIENE."

Butler & Tanner,
The Selwood Printing Works,
Frome, and London.

PREFACE.

WHEN, some years ago, I first undertook the duties of a Medical Officer of Health, I had considerable difficulty in obtaining trustworthy guidance in the preparation of statistical reports. My researches on the subject revealed the fact that the chief if not the only sources of trustworthy information were the official reports of the Registrar-General and some scattered articles in encyclopædias and in the transactions of learned societies. Further investigation showed that, apart from the reports and articles referred to, a large mass of statistical information was current, which was untrustworthy in its methods of compilation and arrangement, and fallacious in its inferences. It became necessary, therefore, to enter on a somewhat extensive examination of the whole subject; and from the notes gradually accumulated during the years which have since elapsed, I have prepared the present guide to the subject, in the hope that it may be as useful to others as such a guide would have been to me at an earlier stage.

The issue of the selections from the writings of Dr. Farr ("Vital Statistics") by the Sanitary Institute in 1885, which appeared after I had begun my task, did not prevent me continuing it. Every one interested in the progress of public health owes a debt of gratitude to the Sanitary Institute, and to Mr. N. A. Humphreys, the editor of the work, for thus giving in a readily accessible form these selections from Dr. Farr's writings; but the form in which the work is necessarily cast—consisting of extracts from various reports and articles, the subjects of which not infrequently overlap,—although very valuable for reference, does not meet the requirements of the ordinary student.

It is evident that in such a subject the substantive facts must be derived chiefly from the Registrar-General's Reports; and, where it is not otherwise stated, the reader may assume that the facts adduced in the following pages are derived from this source. The value of the Registrar-General's Reports is increasing year by year; and there is no country in the world which possesses so rich a mine of information for all who know how to avail themselves of its treasures.

Other sources of information are acknowledged in their proper place; and the bibliography on pages xix. to xxi. will indicate the chief authorities which have been consulted in its preparation. I am indebted to my friends, Mr. C. Mansford, B.A., and Mr. W. J. H. Whittall, F.I.A., assistant-actuary to the Clerical, Medical and General Assurance Society, for valuable assistance in the more technical actuarial and mathematical portions of the book.

In conclusion, I venture to hope that this book will be found useful as a guide to junior medical officers of health and to all who are preparing for the various sanitary examinations, whose requirements I have had especially in view in writing it.

ARTHUR NEWSHOLME.

TOWN HALL, BRIGHTON.
March 15*th*, 1889.

PREFACE TO THE SECOND EDITION.

THE fact that a new edition of this book is required within a few months of its first issue is gratifying, as indicating that it meets the needs of students. The opportunity has been taken to make some verbal corrections; but, with these exceptions, the book remains practically as before.

A. N.

TABLE OF CONTENTS.

LIST OF ILLUSTRATIONS.

LIST OF STATISTICAL TABLES.

BIBLIOGRAPHY.

Vital Statistics: A Memorial Volume of Selections from the Reports and Writings of William Farr, M.D., D.C.L., C.B., F.R.S. Edited by N. A. Humphreys, Esq. (Sanitary Institute).

Annual Reports of the Registrar-General of Births, Deaths and Marriages in England for successive years.

Annual Summaries of Births, Deaths and Causes of Death in London and other Great Towns for successive years.

Supplement to the Thirty-fifth Annual Report of the Registrar-General containing the Report of Mortality, 1861–70 (Dr. Farr).

Supplement to the Forty-fifth Annual Report of the Registrar-General containing the Report of Mortality, 1871–80 (Dr. Ogle).

Statistical Reports of the Health of the Navy for successive years.

Statistical Reports of the Health of the Army for successive years.

Fifteenth Annual Report of the Medical Officer to the Local Government Board, 1885–86.

Census of England and Wales, 1881: Preliminary Report.

Census Report, Vol. III., Ages, Conditions as to Marriage, Occupations and Birth-places of the People.

Census Report, Vol. IV., General Report.

Gulstonian Lectures on Medical Statistics, by Dr. F. B. Hawkins (1829).

Principles and Methods of Medical Observation and Research, by Prof. Laycock (1864).

Contributions to Vital Statistics, by F. G. P. Neison (Simpkin, Marshall & Co., 3rd edition, 1857).

On Some Fallacies of Vital Statistics, by Dr. W. H. Rumsey (Smith, Elder & Co., 1875).

Traité de Statistique, by M. Block (Paris, 1878).

An Essay on Probabilities, and on their Application to Life Contingencies and Insurance Offices, by Prof. de Morgan (Longman & Co., 1838).

Principles of Science; Chap. XVII., on the Law of Error, by Prof. Jevons.

Sur l'Homme et le Développement de ses Facultés, par M. A. Quetelet.

Statistics of Families in the Upper and Professional Classes, by Charles Ansell, Jun. (Layton, 1874).

Encyclopedia of Anatomy and Physiology: articles on Medical Statistics and on Vital Statistics, by Dr. W. A. Guy, F.R.S.

On the Importance and Value of Arithmetical Means, by Prof. Radicke (New Sydenham Society, 1861).

The Nomenclature of Diseases, by a Committee of the Royal College of Physicians of London (2nd edition, 1885).

Public Health Reports, by Sir John Simon, F.R.S. Edited by Dr. E Seaton (2 vols.: reprinted by Sanitary Institute).

Treatise on Hygiene and Public Health, by Dr. A. H. Buck. Vol. II. containing article on Statistics (Sampson Low & Co., 1879).

Encyclopœdia Britannica, 8th edition: article on Human Mortality, by Mr. Milne. (This invaluable article is not contained in the 9th edition).

The Value of Death-rates as a Test of Sanitary Condition, by N. A. Humphreys, Esq. (Journal Statistical Society, December, 1874).

The Recent Decline in the English Death-rate, by N. A. Humphreys, Esq. (Journal Statistical Society, June, 1883).

The Recent Decline in the English Death-rate, considered in connection with the Causes of Death, by Dr. G. B. Longstaff (Journal Statistical Society, June, 1884).

The Effect of Migration in Disturbing Local Rates of Mortality, by D. A. Welton, Esq. (16th vol. Journal of Society of Actuaries, 1871).

Some Aspects of Mortality Statistics, by Dr. L. Parkes (Public Health, 1888).

Figures, Facts, and Fallacies, by Dr. E. F. Willoughby (San. Record, 1884).

The Mutual Relations of the Birth-rate and Death-rate, by Dr. Bristowe, F.R.S. (St. Thomas's Hospital Reports, Vol. VII., 1876).

A Paper on Some of the Defects in the Present System of Registration of Deaths in England and Wales, by Dr. A. Ransome, F.R.S. (Social Science Congress, 1867).

Losses and Gains in the Death-toll of England and Wales during the last thirty years, by Dr. Ransome (Philosophical Society, Manchester, 1876).

On Some of the Numerical Tests of the Health of Towns, by Dr. Ransome (1863).

On the Form of the Epidemic Wave, and Some of its Probable Causes, by Dr. Ransome (Trans. Epidemiological Society, 1881–2).

On the Vital Statistics of Towns, by Dr. Ransome (Manchester Statistical Society, 1888).

On the Ticketed Houses of Glasgow, by Dr. J. B. Russell (Glasgow Philosophical Society, 1888).

The Seasonal Prevalence of Continued Fevers in London, by Dr. G. B. Longstaff (Trans. Epidemiological Society, 1885).

On the Number of Deaths from Accident, Negligence, Violence, and Misadventure in the United Kingdom and some other Countries, by C. Walford (Stanford, 1881).

Institute of Actuaries Text-book of the Principles of Interest, Life Annuities, and Assurance; Part II., Life Contingencies, by G. King, F.I.A. (Layton, 1887).

A Treatise on the Value of Life Contingencies arranged for the use of Students, by Edward Long, F.R.S.E. (Edinburgh, 1864).

The Doctrine of Life Annuities and Assurances, by Francis Bailey (1813). New Edition with additions (E. Howell, Liverpool, 1864).

Treatise on Annuities, by Griffith Davies, F.R.S. (Layton).

On the Valuation of Annuities and Assurances, by Mr. Milne. 2 vols.

Insurance Handbook and Guide, by C. Walford, F.S.S. (2nd Edition. Layton, 1867).

Mortality Experience of the Prudential Assurance Company for 1867–70 (Layton, 1871).

Institute of Actuaries Life Tables, Tables deduced from the Mortality Experience of Life Assurance Companies, collected and arranged by the Institute of Actuaries (Layton, 1872).

English Life Table, No. 3, by Dr. Farr (Longman & Co., 1864).

INTRODUCTION.

VITAL Statistics may be defined as the science of numbers applied to the life-history of communities and nations; and in the following pages the chief statistical facts concerning the various phases and stages of life will be in turn presented. The subject naturally divides itself into two sections: first, the sources of information, as the census enumerations, registration of births, marriages, sickness, death, etc.; and second, the information derived from these sources, which will be discussed in detail in the following pages. (See table of contents, pages ix.–xiii.).

As the scope of a science widens, it is generally found necessary sooner or later to adopt numerical standards of comparison. In medical science this is found to be especially necessary, though perhaps in no other science is the difficulty of exact numerical statement so great. The value of *experience*, founded on an accumulation of individual facts, varies greatly according to the character of the observer. As Dr. Guy has put it: "The *sometimes* of the cautious is the *often* of the sanguine, the *always* of the empiric, and the *never* of the sceptic; while the numbers 1, 10, 100, 10,000, have but one meaning for all mankind."

The variable accuracy of individual observers makes us distrustful of generalities founded on imperfect reasoning or defective facts, and necessitates the use of figures. Experience tells us that a certain event is to be expected, while the numerical method can tell us how often it is to be expected. We shall discuss later on the application of the numerical method to medical problems, and the difficulties involved in it. It is sometimes said *that statistics may be made to prove anything;* and no doubt they may be manipulated in such a manner as to make it difficult to detect the fallacies involved in their abuse. But this ignorant or unscrupulous abuse of figures does not discredit their legitimate use, and that they have a very important and perfectly trustworthy application to medical facts will be abundantly shown in the following pages; while at the same time we hope to effectually guard against the errors which many writers have committed, and so help to rescue the subject from that disrepute into which it has undeservedly fallen.

VITAL STATISTICS.

CHAPTER I.

POPULATION.

Requirements of Correct Statistics.—Census Enumerations.—Age and Sex Grouping of Population.—Criticism of Accuracy of Census.—Methods of Estimating Population.—Registrar-General's Official Method.—Instances of Mistaken Estimates.—Estimation from Number of Inhabited Houses.—Estimation from Birth-rate.—Quinquennial Census.—Requirements of a good Census.—Effect of Migration on Population.—Population Registers.—Progress of Population.—Economic Value of Population.

TO obtain correct vital statistics, it is essential to have (1) a correct enumeration of the population; (2) a complete and accurate registration of births and deaths and other important events in the life-history of individuals, as marriages and sickness; and (3) an accurate statement of the age, sex, and cause of death of each deceased person.

An accurate estimate of **population** is the first desideratum, for population forms the natural basis of all vital statistics. In comparing different communities, it is necessary to state the deaths and other statistical data in terms of the population otherwise no true comparison can be instituted.

The actual population is known only by census enumerations For the years intervening between two census enumerations estimates of the population are made.

The first **census** of modern times was taken in the year 1751 in Sweden. In this country the first census was in 1801, and then decennially, the ninth being taken on April 4th, 1881. The first census, in 1801, showed the number of males and females of each house and family, and the occupation, classified roughly as agricultural, trading, and others not comprised under these two heads. In 1821 information was first sought as to ages, but it was left optional whether this information should be furnished or not. The first census which could be described as fairly complete was that of 1851, which was organized under Dr. Farr's supervision. It obtained information as to occupation, birthplace, relationship (husband, wife, etc.), civil condition (married, widow, bachelor, etc.), and the number of persons deaf and dumb or blind. At this census, under the powers given by the Census Act, the precise age at last birthday of each person in the country was first demanded. The accuracy of the information under this head has been impugned; but it is noteworthy that the mean age of females as returned in England exceeds the mean age of males by ten months, so that the tendency of women to understate their ages evidently only operates in comparatively small numbers.

In the census report of 1881 the age and sex distribution of the population of each urban and rural sanitary authority, as constituted that year, was given for the first time. It is now, therefore, possible in these large districts and towns to give the death-rate at each group of ages and in the two sexes separately, a result which, as we shall subsequently find, is of the highest importance (p. 101).

Dr. Farr, many years ago, found that in both the death registers and the census schedules there was a tendency for the ages to be stated in round numbers, as 30, 40, 50, etc. In classifying ages, he therefore adopted the groups 25–35, 35–45, etc., which minimises the effect of such displacement of ages. It would be well if all medical officers of health would adopt the same groups of ages in their annual reports, as comparison of results would be thus rendered possible.

The correctness of census enumerations has been doubted chiefly on three grounds: (1) the infrequency of the census; and (2) the consequent incompetence of the enumerators; and (3) misrepresentations of the enumerated, either from ignorance or wilful misrepresentation. We have already alluded to inaccuracy in respect of information as to *age*. Such errors are most apt to occur at the extremes of age. They are of greatest importance in the first years of life, infants being often returned in the census a year older than their true age. The methods of checking these errors will be subsequently described. *Infirmities* are apt, for obvious reasons, to be understated.

The most serious error, however, occurs in regard to *occupations*. Master and servant are confused. Thus a watchmaker may mean either the master or a journeyman; and there are similar errors arising from the fact that of those returned under a given occupation, some are actually engaged in it, while others have retired from it.

Each succeeding census, however, is more accurate and complete, and with the advance of education among the masses of the people, the information obtained will become still more reliable.

Estimates of Population require to be made in the intervals between each census and the next succeeding one. Several methods of varying accuracy have been proposed.

1. Theoretically, if we knew the number of births and deaths, and of emigrants and immigrants since the last census, the population in any year could be accurately stated. But an uncertain number of births and a smaller number of deaths escape registration, and although the number of emigrants is roughly known, there is no information as to the number of immigrants into this country.

2. It is assumed that *the increase of population* in an established country like ours *remains fairly constant* from one decade to another. Thus, given the population of any town or district in April, 1871 and 1881, and required to find the population, say, in the middle of 1888. The difference between the two census populations divided by 10 will, on this supposition, give the annual increase of population, and this multiplied by the number of years since 1881, and added on to the population of 1881, will give the total population in April, 1888. In estimating death and other rates of a non-stationary population, the *mean population* of the year must be taken. For the three months between April and June, 1888, therefore, add on one-fourth of the annual increase of population.

Thus,—

$$\frac{\text{Popul}^{n}.\text{ in 1881} - \text{Popul . in 1871}}{10} = \text{annual increase of popul}^{n}.$$

$$\text{Annual increase} \times 7 + \frac{\text{annual increase}}{4} + \text{population in 1881} = \text{mean population in 1888.}$$

For example,—

If population in 1871=32,000, and the population in 1881 =36,000, what is the mean population in 1885?

$$\frac{36{,}000-32{,}000}{10} = 400 = \text{annual increase.}$$

$$\frac{400}{4} = 100 = \text{increase from Easter to Midsummer.}$$

$$400 \times 4 + 100 + 36{,}000 = \underline{37{,}700} = \text{mean population of 1885.}$$

This method of estimating the population, which assumes that the annual increase of population throughout a decade is constant in each year, is necessarily fallacious, as it makes no allowance for the increased number of parents year by year, owing to steadily increasing numbers who year by year attain marriageable years. The error is similar to the assumption that simple interest and compound interest will produce identical results. In simple interest the principal remains constant, and a constant rate of interest would produce a constant actual increase in capital. With compound interest, however, the capital (by addition of principal and interest) becomes greater each year, and consequently the interest itself increases year by year. In other words, with compound interest the rate of interest remains the same, but the principal on which the interest is calculated is increased year by year.

3. The *Registrar-General's method* is based on the assumption that the same *rate of increase* will hold good as in the previous intercensal period.

In order to show how this principle is applied, we have to consider the following problem, which, it will be seen, is practically the same as a problem in compound interest, and demands for its treatment an elementary knowledge of the principles of logarithms, which can be obtained from the introduction to any table of logarithms, or from any standard work on algebra.

Having given the population of a district at any fixed date, to find the population a given number of years hence.

Now the extent to which the population will have increased will clearly depend upon the annual rate of increase; *i.e.*, the rate per cent. or per unit by which the births exceed the deaths in the population in question.

Suppose, for the sake of example, that this net annual rate of increase is r per unit of population, so that for every unit at the beginning of the year there exists $1+r$ at the end of that year, or, which is the same thing, there exists $1+r$ of population at the beginning of the second year. Then assuming that the *same rate of increase* continues in the second year, the population at the end of that year will be found by the following proposition:

$1:1+r::1+r:(1+r)^2$=population at end of second year.

Similarly $1:1+r::(1+r)^2:(1+r)^3$=population at end of third year.

In like manner the population at the end of the nth year will on the same principles be $(1+r)^n$, the formula being precisely the same as in compound interest when r=interest of one pound per annum.

From these formulæ, which give the results for every unit of population at the end of one, two, three, etc., n years to be $(1+r)^1, (1+r)^2, (1+r)^3 \quad . \quad . \quad . \quad (1+r)^n$, we easily find the corresponding formulæ for population P. For if we commence with population P, then, since every unit in n years produces $(1+r)^n$, the total result will be P times $(1+r)^n=P(1+r)^n$. By giving to n the successive values 1, 2, 3, etc., we obtain the population produced by P after 1, 2, 3, etc., years.

It will simplify these formulæ if we write $R=1+r$.

Then a population of P will, after n years, amount to $P(1+r)^n = PR^n$, where R = *amount* of every unit of population in one year, the word amount being used as in the language of interest, to represent the original unit + the increase for one year = principal and interest added together.

Now in order to apply these formulæ to any given population it will be first requisite to find the value of r. This may be done if we know the population at any two consecutive census enumerations in the following way. Let P=population at the one census, and P′=population at the next census following. Then if r=annual rate of increase per unit, and $R=1+r$=annual amount of each unit per annum, it is clear from what has been already shown that

$$P(1+r)^n=PR^n=P'.$$

But $n=10$ in this case.

$\therefore$ $PR^{10}=P'$. Hence taking the log. of each side of this equation,

Log. P + 10 log. R = log. P′, and

10 log. R = log. P′ − log. P.

$\therefore$ log. R $=\frac{1}{10}$ (log. P′ − log. P)

Whence R is easily obtained from a table of logs.

An example will make this clear.

If the census population of a town is 32,000 in 1871, and 36,000 in 1881, what is the mean population in 1885?

Here P=32,000, P′=36,000.

Hence log. P′ = log. 36,000 = 4·556303.

And log. P = log. 32,000 = 4·505150.

$\therefore$ log. P′ − log. P = 0·051153.

And $\frac{1}{10}$ (log. P′ − log. P) = 0·005115 = log. R = log. $(1+r)$.

$\therefore$ R, *i.e.* $1+r=1{\cdot}0118$ from the tables.

Also $n=1885\frac{1}{2}-1881\frac{1}{4}=4\frac{1}{4}$ years.

We take $1885\frac{1}{2}$, because the mean population is the population at the middle of the year; and $1881\frac{1}{4}$ because the census was taken in April, 1881.

Therefore in this case

$P'=PR^n$, where P=36,000, R=1·0118, and $n=4\frac{1}{4}$.

$\therefore$ P′ = population required $=36{,}000\times(1{\cdot}0118)^{\frac{17}{4}}$.

And log. P′ = log. 36,000 + $\frac{17}{4}$ log. 1·0118.

But log. 1·0118 = 0·005115.

$\therefore\ \frac{17}{4}$ log. 1·0118=0·021739 }
And log. 36,000 =4·556303 }
Consequently by addition log. P′=4·578042.

And from tables P′=37,848, the required population of 1885.

The assumption that the same rate of increase holds good as in the previous decade is by no means universally true. A population may remain stationary, or even decline; or, on the other hand, may increase very rapidly, from the rise of some new industry, or by reason of a place becoming notorious as a health resort. Thus (*Lancet*, August, 1888) the estimated population of Bradford in the middle of 1888 was 229,721, but there is a note in the Registrar-General's weekly returns, that, judging by the number of houses in the rate-books, there are grounds for believing that the population is over-estimated, and, therefore, the death-rate under-estimated. In the year 1881, the birth-rate in Bradford was 33·0 per 1,000 inhabitants, but in 1887, on the Registrar-General's hypothesis, it was only 27·7, which in a manufacturing town is so low as to suggest some error. The calculated birth-rate of England and Wales fell from 33·9 in 1881 to 31·4 in 1887, but even in the improbable event of the Bradford birth-rate falling in the same proportion it would be only 30·6. If the true birth-rate was 30·6 in Bradford in 1887, then the corresponding population was only 202,712 instead of 224,507, as published by the Registrar-General. If 202,712 was the true population, then the death-rate in 1887 was 22·0 instead of 19·9, and the zymotic death-rate similarly was 3·16 instead of 2·86 per 1,000 inhabitants.

It is evident from this example that the Registrar-General's method may in individual cases allow the possibility of an error of at least 10 per cent. With such an error a recorded death-rate of 20 per 1,000 may represent an actual death-rate of 18 or of 22 per 1,000.

Other examples are given in the *Sanitary Record* of September, 1888. Thus

In 1881 the population of Paddington was estimated at 123,677; the census showed it to be 107,218.

In 1881 the population of Kensington was estimated at 206,422; the census showed it to be 163,151.

In 1881 the population of Hampstead was estimated at 54,541; the census showed it to be 45,452.

In these cases the estimated numbers were 15·25 and 20 per cent. respectively over the actual numbers, so that a death-rate of 15 per 1,000 in Kensington on the assumed population was one of 18·75 on the actual population. At the 1871 census the population of Gosport was found to have been over-estimated to the extent of 33 per cent., and of Cambridge under-estimated by about 15 per cent. Dr. Longstaff, in a letter to the *Times* in August, 1888, maintains that there are strong reasons for believing that the total population of the United Kingdom is half a million less than the official estimate. The Registrar-General in his 50th Annual Report shows, however, that although the birth-rate in the last few years has decreased, the death-rate has decreased to a corresponding extent, and although emigration has increased, an increased immigration has been proved by Mr. Giffen to accompany increased emigration, and that there is reason to believe, therefore, that the official estimate of the population of England and Wales is moderately accurate. At the same time, this does not obviate the inaccuracies resulting from the application of the official method to the different districts and towns of the country.

4. The results obtained by the previous methods may be to some extent checked by ascertaining *the number of inhabited houses* for the year from the assessment books, and then multiplying this by the average number of inhabitants in each house, as ascertained at the last census. This method, although it forms a useful check on the preceding method, involves the fallacy that new houses may be of a different class from those previously in existence, and may therefore have a different number of occupants. In the rapidly growing suburbs of London, where old-fashioned large houses with gardens have been superseded by terraces of small houses, this is particularly the case; but in many instances this method gives an approximately correct result.

In Brighton, in 1861, the number of inhabited houses was 12,727, of persons, 77,693, equal to nearly 6·1 persons per house. Now in 1871 the number of inhabited houses was 14,438, and at the same rate the population should have been 88,071 instead of 90,011, the actual number. The difference was probably due in great measure to the increased number of large hotels.

It should be noted also that there is often difficulty in ascertaining from officials the number of inhabited houses for the current year. An estimate founded on previous years is, of course, open to all the fallacies connected with similar estimates of population.

5. An additional means of checking the official population is obtained, if we assume that the *birth-rate per* 1,000 *inhabitants remains fairly constant* in a series of years. On this assumption, the number of births in any year being registered, the population is easily calculated.

Thus in the Wandsworth District the average birth-rate for the ten years 1872–81 was 35·68 per 1,000, and the number of births in 1881 was 7,582. Therefore the population in 1881, on the assumption that 35·68 was the birth-rate, was

$$\frac{7582 \times 1000}{35{\cdot}68} = 212{,}500$$

By the census return the population in 1881 was found to be 210,434, to which a small addition must be made for increase during the second quarter of the census year.

By finding the estimated population of the Wandsworth District in 1881, according to the Registrar-General's method, we can compare the accuracy of the results obtained by the two methods.

Population of Wandsworth District in 1861 was 70,403, and in 1871 was 125,050.

Required to estimate the population in 1881.

By adopting the method described on p. 6 it will be found to be 221,093, much further remote from the facts as revealed by the census than the population estimated from the birth-rate. It should be remembered that the birth-rate started with has been calculated on the Registrar-General's official estimate of the population; and the preceding method can therefore only be regarded as testing the consistency of his figures, and not as determining the actual population.

The conclusion from the preceding discussion on estimates of population is, that a more frequent census is required. Every calculation in vital statistics rests on the assumption that the population is accurately known, and consequently the trustworthiness of such calculations steadily diminishes as the interval from the preceding census increases.

It must be remembered that the *mean population* of the year is taken as the basis of calculation of mortality and other rates, which involves an estimate, even in the census year, for the three months between the census and midsummer. It would therefore be advantageous to have the census enumerations at the end of June as well as to have them more frequently.

A Quinquennial Census would go far to remedy the present uncertainties. Such a census is practised in France and Germany (triennial in some German states), in New Zealand, Queensland, Manitoba, and the North-western Territory of Canada, as well as in twelve states and three territories of the American republic. It is true that there are not as powerful reasons for a quinquennial census as on the continent, where it is required for military purposes; nor is there the same necessity as in many American states, where the increment of population is by leaps and bounds, and not steadily, as in most parts of our own country. Still, however, there are very strong reasons why a quinquennial census should be adopted.

Vital statistics must always furnish the basis on which sanitary reforms shall rest, especially in regard to legislation. Dr. Farr may in this sense be called the father of sanitary science. There are also political reasons for the change, as political representation for both imperial and local purposes will rest in future on a strictly numerical basis. In addition, a more frequent census would lead to the work being better done, owing to less difficulty in collecting a sufficient staff of intelligent enumerators, and greater experience on their part. The chief obstacle is the expense of the enumeration; but in view of the important results obtainable, it may be hoped that the reform will be soon realized. The Government has been recently memorialised on the subject by the Statistical Society, and a deputation urging its importance has been favourably received by the Secretary of the Local Government Board (Dec., 1888).

The **Requirements of a good Census** from a sanitarian's standpoint are, that the enumeration shall be accurate and complete, and that it shall be rapid and simultaneous throughout the country, in order to avoid the disturbing influences of migration. The particulars stated should comprise the following items as a minimum: name, sex, age (children under two years stated in months), relation to head of household, conjugal condition, calling, religious persuasion, illiteracy, birthplace and nationality, language, residence, infirmities. The occupation should be given with such definition as will obviate confusion, and will enable different classes to be compared. The accurate enumeration of age and sex is of great importance, as on it depends the correct interpretation of mortality statistics.

Effect of Migration on Population.—Between any two censuses there is a constant inflow and outflow of population. There is first the *natural increment* of population due to the excess of births over deaths. Then there is the inflow caused by the presence in this country of visitors and settlers from other countries; while there is the much larger outflow due to the departure of travellers and emigrants. Probably there is no other State in Europe in which the influence of immigration and emigration is so great as in England. In the ten years 1871–80 the natural increment of the population was 3,425,982, the actual increment (as determined by the census) was 3,256,020. Thus in ten years there was a loss by excess of emigration over immigration of 169,962, which excess consisted of 138,324 males and 31,638 females.

Population Registers.—The only way in which an exact record of migration can be kept is by *population registers*, which are kept in Sweden, Belgium, Holland, and Italy. The number of emigrants from England and Wales is approximately known from the annual returns of the Board of Trade, but there are no trustworthy data as to immigration.

During the year 1886 there were in England and Wales 903,866 births and 537,276 deaths, so the natural increment was 366,590, equal to 1·32 per cent of the estimated population at the beginning of the year. Now the population of England and Wales enumerated in April, 1881, was 25,974,439 persons. The excess of births over deaths (natural increment) from that date to the middle of 1886 was 1,971,600, making the population in 1886, if determined simply by natural increment, 27,946,039. We have no data, however, for checking the influence of migration, and are obliged, therefore, to assume the same rate of increase as in the previous intercensal period, on which assumption the population of England and Wales in the middle of 1886 consisted of 27,870,586 persons.

Migration not only affects the actual numbers of persons, but has an important effect on the age and sex of the resultant population. Inasmuch as the mortality differs in the two sexes and at different ages, it is evidently of great importance to know for statistical purposes the age and sex constitution of a population.

Progress of Population.—The following table shows the population of England and Wales and London at each of the nine census enumerations:

Census Year.	Population of	
	England and Wales.	London.
1801	8,892,536	958,863
1811	10,164,256	1,138,815
1821	12,000,236	1,378,947
1831	13,896,797	1,654,994
1841	15,914.148	1,948,417
1851	17,927,609	2,362,236
1861	20,066,224	2,803,989
1871	22,712,266	3,254,260
1881	25,968,286	3,814,571

Thus in England every 100 persons living in 1801 had increased to 132 in 1821, and every 100 persons living in 1821 had increased to 132 in 1841. Every 100 persons living in 1801 had increased to 175 in 1841, and at the same rate of increase would amount to 200 in the year 1850 and to 300 in the year 1879. The mean rate of increase was ·0141 per unit, or 1·41 per cent. annually during these years. The method by which these facts are worked out is as follows :—

Let r = rate of increase per unit of population, so that
$1+r$ = population at end of one year; and generally
$(1+r)^n$ = „ „ „ n years.
Let $R=(1+r)$
Then if P = total population in any given year.
n = number of years under observation.
P′ = population at end of n years.
$$P\,(1+r)^n=PR^n=P'$$

To find the time in which a population will double itself, *i.e.* in which P′ will become equal to 2 P.

$$P'=PR^n$$
$$2\,P=PR^n$$
$$\therefore R^n=2$$
$$n \log R=\log 2$$
$$n=\frac{\log 2}{\log R}=\frac{\log 2}{\log (1+r)}$$
= number of years in which the population doubles itself.

In the preceding instance $r=\cdot0141$.

$$\therefore n=\frac{\log 2}{\log 1\cdot0141}=\frac{\cdot3010300}{\cdot0060808}=49\cdot5 \text{ years.}$$

Similarly, to find in how many years the population trebles itself, we have—

$$n=\frac{\log 3}{\log 1\cdot0141}=\frac{\cdot4771213}{\cdot0060808}=78\cdot4 \text{ years.}$$

The following table gives the estimated population and the area of the United Kingdom, and its several portions in the middle of 1886 :—

	Persons.	Males.	Females.	Area in Acres.
United Kingdom .	36,709,477	17,871,248	18,838,289	77,143,938
England and Wales	27,870,586	13,562,621	14,307,965	37,239,351
Scotland	3,949,393	1,911,997	2,037,396	19,084,659
Ireland	4,889,498	2,396,630	2,492,868	20,819,928

Economic Value of Population.—Dr. Farr has shown that each individual member of the community has an actual money value represented by the wages he is capable of earning, and that this constitutes the most important factor in the wealth of the community. Deducting the amount required for subsistence, £150 is the mean net value of each member of the male population estimated by the standard of the agricultural labourer. This amount is obtained by capitalizing the income derived from wages and deducting all the expenses of subsistence. It is evident that this value will vary greatly at different ages, being partly dependent upon the expectation of life, and very low in infancy on account of the high death-rate under five years of age. On Dr. Farr's basis, the child of an agricultural labourer is worth only £5 at birth, £56 at the age of 5, £117 at the age of 10, £192 at the age of 15, increasing to £246 at the age of 25, then steadily declining to only £1 at the age of 70, while at 80 the cost of future maintenance is greater than the earnings by £41. It is evident that diseases like enteric fever and phthisis, which destroy life at its most productive period, must necessarily involve an immense waste of money, and that the economic value of the population has been increased by sanitary measures. Thus by Dr. Farr's English Life Table the mean lifetime is 40·86 years; by the Healthy Districts Life Table it is 49·0 years. It is fair to assume that if the mean lifetime in the latter case is one-fifth greater than in the former, at least one-fifth has been added to the money value of a working population.

CHAPTER II.

REGISTRATION OF BIRTHS AND DEATHS.

History of Registration.—System of Registration.—Defects of Registration.—Number of Uncertified Deaths.—Number of Inquests.—Improvements of Registration required.—Medical Registrars.—Registration of Causes of Death.—Deaths from ill-defined Causes.—Lack of Uniformity of Nomenclature.—Classification of Diseases.—The Royal College of Physicians on Nomenclature and Classification.—The Registrar-General's Classification of Causes of Death.

NEXT to a correct enumeration of population, the accurate and complete registration of births, marriages, and deaths constitutes an essential basis of vital statistics. The question of registration of disease will be discussed in the next chapter.

Such is the importance of this matter, that the late Dr. Parkes only expresses the literal truth when he says: "The attention now paid to public health is in a large degree owing to the careful collection of the statistics of births and deaths, and of the causes of death, made in England during the last forty years. It may truly be said, indeed, that not only all Europe, but gradually the entire world, has been influenced by the work of the Registrar-General of England. We are now able to determine with some precision the limits of mortality and its causes, and are being led up to the consideration of the causes which bring about a high death-rate."

History of Registration. — The office of Registrar-General of England was created in 1836, and civil registration began as the result of an Act of Parliament on July 1st, 1837. The first of the series of annual reports of the Registrar-General was published in 1839, and to this first report Dr. W. Farr, who acted as Compiler of Abstracts in the newly created General Register Office, contributed the first of that long series of letters, addressed to the Registrar-General, on the causes of death in England, which have become so widely known, and must be constantly referred to by all who write on Vital Statistics. Even in this first letter he emphasized the importance of a correct and exact medical momenclature, saying that "the nomenclature is of as much importance in this department of inquiry as weights and measures in the physical sciences." Successive amendments to the law of registration were made, and in 1874 a new law was enacted, rendering the registration of births and deaths compulsory, with penalties for non-compliance.

In the 39½ years before registration became compulsory, the registration of births was defective, the proportion of unregistered births being estimated at about 5 per cent. Only a small proportion of deaths were believed to have escaped registration, though in a considerable proportion the medical certificate of cause of death was either unsatisfactory or altogether wanting. The returns of 1876 showed the excellent effect of the compulsory law. The stated birth-rate of that year, 36·6 per thousand, was the highest on record, being 1·2 per thousand higher than the average for the ten previous years; while the number of uncertified deaths had greatly decreased.

System of Registration. — The registration of births and of deaths is performed either at the offices of local registrars or the houses of the people. Copies of the certificates are forwarded to the General Register Office, Somerset House, where they are collated and abstracted; and from these abstracts the weekly, quarterly, and annual reports of the Registrar-General are prepared. For the twenty-eight great English towns a weekly report is issued on the Tuesday morning next following the end of the week, which contains fuller information in regard to the causes of death in London, and states also the death-rate in the principal foreign towns, as well as the meteorological facts of the week. The quarterly reports for

England and Wales are issued in the month following the end of the quarter, while the annual reports appear toward the end of the year subsequent to the year to which they apply. An annual summary, however, appears at an earlier date, and in regard to the delay in the issue of the annual reports, it must be remembered that they are works of much labour and skill, and necessarily occupy considerable time in preparation. As Dr. Farr says: "They may be regarded as storehouses of facts, which have been arranged on methods that are approved as the most useful and convenient, and to which, both now and in future years, students of vital statistics may resort for the elucidation of questions bearing on the social condition of the people, on national progress, on life, health, and disease. It is important they should be *done well.* It is desirable only in the next degree that they should be *done quickly.*"

The admirable decennial supplements of Dr. Farr have been continued since his decease by Dr. Ogle, and we shall have frequently to refer to their contents.

The value of these various reports can scarcely be exaggerated. The rates of mortality in the weekly reports require, however, to be accepted with caution, as large fluctuations in short periods may be due to accidental causes. But in indicating the character and amount of prevalent diseases, and their geographical distribution, they are invaluable. As Farr eloquently puts it: "Thus observers, like watchmen on the walls, are ever on the look out, so that they can see exactly what is going on, and neither plague, cholera, nor any other great epidemic can take the nations by surprise. The deaths serve the purpose of a self-registering inspection. Death cannot be deceived by sham defences."

Imperfections of Registration.—In order that registration may have its full value, the facts should be given uniformly, accurately, and completely. There are imperfections in the present system of registration, which are, however, steadily diminishing in extent and importance.

1. A certain proportion of the *births remain unregistered.* (*a*) There is strong reason for thinking that a certain number

of children born alive are buried as *still-born*. (*b*) In addition to these, a small proportion of births escape registration from negligence; in other cases (*c*) owing to the shame of illegitimacy, especially in large towns; others (*d*) in order to avoid compulsory vaccination; and also (*e*) among migratory people, as gypsies, Italians, etc. The Act of 1837 made registration voluntary on the part of the parent, saying he shall give information when requested to do so by the local registrar, but there being no penalty for refusal. Spite of this deficiency in the law, the number of unregistered births steadily decreased. The estimate of the annual deficiency in births registered during 1861–70 (founded on the Census Report) was 13,614 out of 763,623, as compared with an annual deficiency of 19,323 in 1851–60, and of 38,036 in the years 1841–50.

2. The *registration of deaths*, both as regard the fact itself and the cause of death, is steadily becoming more satisfactory, as will be shown shortly. There is still, however, a possibility of deaths escaping registration. In my annual report (1884) as Medical Officer of Health for Clapham, I made the following remarks, which refer to this point. "An important defect of the Registration of Deaths Act may be here alluded to. It is not necessary to register the death of any person before burial, but the 17th section of 37 and 38 Vict., cap. 58, provides that the person who buries or performs any religious service for the burial of any dead body as to which no order or certificate under this section is delivered to him, shall within seven days after the burial give notice thereof to the registrar, and if he fail to do so shall be liable to a fine not exceeding £10. In the case which drew attention to this defect in the Act, the parents, who were unmarried, only lived two days in this subdistrict before their child died. They then took the body to Chelsea, obtained a death certificate from a medical man who had previously known the child, and subsequently buried the child at Hanwell. A week after the burial, and two weeks after the death, a misdirected *postcard* was received by the Clapham registrar from the person who officiated at the burial, baldly stating this fact. It is evident that such a conjunction

of circumstances renders evasion of investigation in suspicious cases a comparatively easy task."

Number of Uncertified Deaths.—In 1886 the causes of 490,264, or 91·3 per cent., of the total deaths were certified by registered medical practitioners; while the causes of 28,690, or 5·3 per cent., were certified by coroners; and the causes of 18,322, or 3·4 per cent. of the total deaths, were not certified. In the previous years the proportion of uncertified deaths had steadily declined from 4·7 per cent. in 1879 to 3·5 per cent. in 1885. The number of uncertified deaths varies greatly in different parts of the country. Thus in 1886 the proportion in the metropolis was only 1·1 per cent., while in Durham it was 5·6, in Cornwall and Huntingdonshire 6·0, in Herefordshire 6·3 and in Wales 8·1 per cent.

Proportion per 100 *Deaths of Uncertified Deaths.*

	1880.	1881.	1882.	1883.	1884.	1885.
England and Wales . .	4·3	4·1	3·9	3·7	3·6	3·5
Wales	11·4	11·0	10·4	9·3	9·6	8·5
Cornwall	8·7	7·0	6·9	6·6	6·6	5·9
Wiltshire	1·3	0·8	1·1	0·7	0·7	0·8
Durham	7·2	7·2	6·9	5·8		5·8
London	1·3	1·3	1·2	1·3	1·1	1·3

A considerable proportion of these uncertified deaths were submitted by the registrars to the coroner, who in an informal manner decided that no inquest was required. Such a procedure would be justifiable if a private medical investigation were instituted, but as matters now stand there is little reason to doubt that many crimes remain undetected, which investigation would have brought to light. Even when a coroner's inquest is held, the result is often little if at all more satisfactory.

Number of Inquests.—During the year 1886, 28,690 inquests were held; *i.e.*, on 5·3 per cent of the total deaths, the proportion having varied in the seven preceding years from

4·9 to 5·5 per cent. The death on account of which an inquest is held is very commonly registered subsequently as "from natural causes," the coroner considering his sole function to be the detection of crime, and ignoring entirely the medical problems toward the solution of which he might contribute so greatly. In other inquest cases the certification is almost equally defective, the cause of death being returned as "sudden death," "death by the visitation of God," "found dead," etc. Such returns are useless for classification; and it goes almost without saying that no coroner's inquest is satisfactory which does not include a post-mortem examination by a competent medical practitioner.

Improvements in Registration required.—This unsatisfactory state of matters would be effectually remedied by the adoption of the system advocated by Dr. Farr as early as 1864. As matters now stand, when there is no medical certificate of the cause of death, the registrar makes inquiries of the relatives of the deceased person, and if he is satisfied with their explanation of the cause of death, enters it according to their statements, adding the statement that the death is "not medically certified." If he does not care to undertake the responsibility he refers the matter to the coroner, who generally gets his officer, a functionary as irresponsible as the local registrar, to make inquiries. If the coroner's officer reports favourably, the coroner writes to the registrar that an inquest is unnecessary. Such a system is obviously open to the grossest abuses. All this would be remedied if, as Dr. Farr proposed, *medical registrars* were appointed, who should be in close association with the local sanitary authority, and whose duty it would be to inquire into the causes of death where there was no certificate or an unsatisfactory cause of death was returned.

The medical officer of health ought to be the medical registrar of each district, and it should be part of his duty to make a medical inquisition into the cause of death in all dubious cases.

At the present time every medical practitioner is required under a penalty to certify the causes of his patients' death. Such compulsory certification under a penalty cannot be justified in the absence of remuneration. The medical practitioner should receive a fee for his certificate, and the certificate should never come into the hands of the relatives of the deceased person, but be sent direct to the local registrar. This would insure much more accurate results, as at present family practitioners have great difficulty in returning the true cause of death in cases of alcoholism, syphilis, etc.

The Registration of Causes of Death has given an immense impetus to sanitary work, and it is scarcely too much to say that modern sanitary science owes its existence to the registration of deaths and their causes, and the localization of insanitary conditions thereby insured. By its means we are able to submit to numerical analysis the facts relating to the laws of vitality, the influence of age and sex, of civilization, occupation, locality, season, and many other agencies; and our knowledge of all the facts bearing on health and disease has attained a precision never before known.

There are certain **fallacies** in the registration of causes of death, partly owing to the imperfection of medical science and of a portion of its practitioners, and partly owing to differences of nomenclature and classification of diseases.

The deaths uncertified have been already considered. It is evident that as these gradually diminish there will be a transference to death under some definite head. The same applies to the mortality from ill-defined causes, the increased accuracy of diagnosis causing a steady decrease under this head. Thus in 1886 there were 29,283 deaths classed as from "*ill-defined and not specified causes*," being 5·5 per cent of the total deaths. In 1862 the death-rate in England and Wales per million living was 2,104 under this head; in 1872 it was 1,854; and in 1882 it was 1,154, decreasing still further to 1,047 per million living in 1886.

The number in 1886 would have been greater had not between two and three thousand letters been sent out from the Registrar-General's office (a system first started in 1881, when about 1,200 letters of inquiry were sent) to medical men, asking for further information than was given in their certificates.

The information received in answer to these inquiries reduced the deaths under dropsy from 966 to 336, adding the balance to cardiac renal and hepatic diseases. Similarly an addition was made of 202 deaths to childbirth and puerperal fever, of 148 deaths to violence, and of 472 deaths to other headings.

Faulty diagnosis, and the desire to shield relatives, are perhaps the most prolific sources of inaccurate and indefinite certificates. In many cases the certified causes of death are, as Dr. Rumsey long ago pointed out, nothing more than *modes* of death, as cardiac syncope. The most common headings found in this indefinite class are, *abdominal disease*, *debility*, *atrophy*, *inanition*, *innutrition*, *wasting*, *congenital debility*, *cachexia*, *tumour*, *blood-poisoning*, *hæmorrhage*, *dropsy*, *convulsions*, etc.

Peritonitis standing alone is similarly unsatisfactory without its cause being defined, a large proportion of the cases being puerperal in origin.

In many parts of the country, especially in Wales, the causes of death stated by friends are very commonly accepted by the local registrar, without any medical certificate. This probably explains the prevalence of *consumption* in Wales, any wasting disease, especially if accompanied by cough, being called by that name.

The mortality from "*abdominal disease*" is on the decrease, and this may possibly account for at least a part of the increased mortality in recent years from cancer.

The *lack of uniformity of nomenclature* among medical men is another source of fallacy. There appears to be a fashion even in the names of diseases. In one doctor's practice nearly all the deaths from respiratory diseases will be returned as bronchitis, in another perhaps as pneumonia. It is necessary, therefore, in instituting comparisons for a series of years, to take only some well-marked and easily recognisable cause of death, or some large group of diseases in which the sources of fallacy will counterbalance each other. Such factors do not, however, invalidate the results obtainable from the national statistics. With the exception of the figures relating to alcoholism, syphilis, and perhaps insanity, the figures on the whole are reliable. The case of cancer will be discussed subsequently (page 208). Even the errors themselves tend to balance each other, and are subject to laws which produce more or less constant factors.

Perhaps there is no other case in which variations of nomenclature are so unfortunate as in diphtheria. A large proportion of the deaths due to this disease are doubtless returned as ulcerated throat, quinsy, laryngitis, membranous laryngitis, and especially croup. I have known cases certified as membranous laryngitis which were not entered in the Registrar-General's weekly reports as diphtheria, although they were acknowledged to be this by the practitioner in attendance, when inquiry was made by the local sanitary officials. Croup and quinsy were formerly placed by the Registrar-General next to diphtheria, as zymotic diseases, but have now been relegated to another position in deference to the classification of the Royal College of Physicians, London.

A **perfect medical registration** of causes of death can only be insured by steady and gradual steps. This end will be greatly furthered by,—

(1) Improved education of medical practitioners, especially of those attending the poor, and a development of increased interest on their part in the important results to be obtained from exact statistics.

(2) The appointment of skilled medical sanitarians as local registrars. Such registrars would reject every certificate which was not provided by a qualified person, and would institute further inquiries in dubious cases.

(3) A uniform nomenclature of diseases.

Nomenclature of Diseases.—The necessity of uniformity is obvious, as otherwise any classified results must be untrustworthy. The nomenclature of the Royal College of Physicians of London, of which the second edition and first revision appeared in 1885, is the standard adopted in all English-speaking countries, and all death-returns should be made in accordance with this. Of course no classification will obviate the differences due to the opinions of individual practitioners, as, for instance, the return by one practitioner of death as due to croup which another would certify as diphtheria.

The preface to the R. C. P. classification contains many weighty remarks bearing on this question of **Nomenclature and Classification** which we cannot do better than quote. It is pointed out that the great ends of such a nomenclature are (1) to perfect the statistical registration of diseases, (2) to form a steady basis on which medical experience can be built up, and (3) to throw light on the causes of disease, which, in many cases, may thus be brought within the range of preventibility.

The committee appointed by the Royal College of Physicians expressed their sense of the desirability of as little deviation as possible from the list of names employed by the Registrar-General of England; as otherwise his settled plans and his forms of returns would require to be remodelled, the comparison of future with past returns would be made difficult and perplexing, if not impossible, and a damaging break would be caused in evidence which becomes more and more trustworthy and valuable in proportion as it is prolonged and continuous.

They also refused to exclude names, such as dropsy, palsy, convulsions, merely because they may seem to express only vague or imperfect knowledge, agreeing with Dr. Farr that the refusal to sanction such terms as these in the region of disease "would have an obvious tendency to encourage reckless conjecture" in making returns. The Revision Committee (1885), however, while fully acknowledging the wisdom of the above remark, "felt it right to indicate as strongly as possible the necessity of avoiding the use of the names of symptoms wherever the names of diseases or of causes of symptoms could with reasonable certainty be substituted." Thus the term apoplexy should only be used when the morbid condition causing it cannot be recognised.

The classification of diseases is a more difficult task than their nomenclature, and it is pointed out that the comparison of single diseases (if well marked) is more reliable than that of groups of diseases. But although a good classification is very difficult, it is very important, as it "aids and simplifies the registration of diseases, helps towards a more easy comparison and knowledge of them, and towards the storing of experience respecting them, and facilitates the discovering of general principles from the collected, grouped, and compared phenomena."

A classification might be according to (1) symptoms, (2) causes, (3) intimate nature, (4) tissues or systems of the body affected, (5) parts of the body as they lie anatomically. The committee based their classification on anatomical considerations, and in subservience to this grouped diseases as General and Local. General diseases were divided into section A, comprehending those disorders which appear to involve a morbid condition of the blood, such as the specific fevers; and section B, comprising for the most part disorders which are apt to invade different parts of the same body simultaneously or successively, sometimes called Constitutional Diseases. The Revision Committee pointed out that the name General Diseases fails to express the nature of the group which it heads, and that *Morbi Corporis Universi* would convey more clearly the idea intended, or "Diseases of the whole body and diseases which may be distributed in several parts at one time,—General Diseases."

The system of classification of diseases must *vary according to the object* of the registration. Thus (1) the Registrar-General tabulates deaths and the causes of death. His is essentially a classification based on an etiological basis, and thus possesses a supreme importance from a sanitary standpoint. The College of Physicians' classification is one of diseases, while that of the Registrar-General is of assigned causes of death; one is pathological, the other etiological. This is seen very strikingly in the classification of injuries, the College of Physicians classifying them according to their position and nature, while the Registrar-General divides them into accidental, homicidal, suicidal, and execution.[1]

[1] Similarly cases of whooping cough with death from pneumonia are referred by the Registrar-General to the former and much more remote cause of death. Most classifications which give a single cause of death in their ultimate analysis would ascribe the death to pneumonia.

(2) The army and navy medical departments tabulate diseases as well as deaths occurring in the two services. Hence many diseases appear which are not seen in the death returns.

(3) The registrars of hospitals and the medical officers of infirmaries deal mainly in their returns with the distribution of morbid processes within the body, and seek rather to find the proportion of deaths to attacks than the proportion of number of attacks or deaths to population. As this method takes note of ultimate and proximate causes of deaths, stating the original disease and its complications, there is commonly for each individual disease a multiple return.

It is evident, therefore, that there must co-exist two dissimilar methods of classification, of which the etiological is for our present purposes by far the most important.

Appended is the skeleton of the Registrar-General's classification, as it is on this the details of our knowledge of diseases must be fitted. We must repeat, however, that the knowledge of a separate disease is safer for comparative purposes than that of a group of diseases. For instance, the term Zymotic Diseases includes enteric fever and whooping cough, which certainly have a very unequal value as a test of the sanitary condition of any locality. In regard to constitutional diseases, it should be remembered also that certain diseases, such as contracted granular kidney, which are classed under local diseases, might perhaps more justly come under the head of constitutional diseases, while in other instances the converse holds good.

Registrar-General's Classification of Causes of Death.

I. Specific Febrile or Zymotic Diseases—

1. Miasmatic Diseases—

Smallpox { Vaccinated. / Unvaccinated. / No Statement. }

Chicken Pox.

Measles.

Epidemic Rose Rash.

Scarlet Fever.
Typhus.
Relapsing Fever.
Influenza.
Whooping Cough.
Mumps.
Diphtheria.
Cerebro-Spinal Fever.
Simple and Ill-Defined Fever.
Enteric Fever.
Other Miasmatic Diseases.

2. Diarrhœal Diseases—
Cholera.
Diarrhœa, Dysentery.

3. Malarial Diseases—
Remittent Fever.
Ague.

4. Zoogenous Diseases—
Hydrophobia.
Glanders.
Splenic Fever.
Cowpox and other Effects of Vaccination.

5. Venereal Diseases—
Syphilis.
Gonorrhœa, Stricture of Urethra.

6. Septic Diseases—
Phagedœna.
Erysipelas.
Pyœmia, Septicœmia.
Puerperal Fever.

II. Parasitic Diseases—
Thrush.
Other Diseases from Vegetable Parasites.
Hydatid Disease.
Other Diseases from Animal Parasites

III. Dietetic Diseases—

Starvation, Want of Breast-milk.

Scurvy.

Intemperance { Chronic Alcoholism. / Delirium Tremens. }

IV. Constitutional Diseases—

Rheumatic Fever, Rheumatism of Heart.

Gout.

Rickets.

Cancer.

Tabes Mesenterica.

Tubercular Meningitis (Acute Hydrocephalus).

Phthisis.

Other Forms of Tuberculosis, Scrofula.

Purpura, Hæmorrhagic Diathesis.

Anæmia, Chlorosis, Leucocythœmia.

Diabetes Mellitus.

Other and undefined Constitutional Diseases.

V. Developmental Diseases—

Premature Birth.

Atelectasis.

Cyanosis.

Spina Bifida.

Imperforate Anus.

Cleft Palate, Harelip.

Other Congenital Defects.

Old Age.

VI. Local Diseases—

Diseases of Nervous System.

" " Organs of Special Sense.

" " Circulating System.

" " Respiratory System.

" " Digestive System.

" " Lymphatic System and Ductless Glands.

" " Urinary System.

Diseases of Organs of Generation.
„ „ Parturition.
„ „ Organs of Locomotion.
„ „ Integumentary System.

VII. Violence—

Accident or Negligence.
Homicide
Suicide.
Execution.

VIII. Ill-Defined and Not Specified Causes—

Dropsy.
Debility, Atrophy, Inanition.
Mortification.
Tumour.
Abscess.
Hæmorrhage.
Sudden Deaths (causes unascertained).
Other Ill-defined and Not Specified Causes.

CHAPTER III.

REGISTRATION OF SICKNESS.

Estimation of Prevalence of a Disease from its Mortality.—Economically Sickness more important than Death.—Attempts made to Register Sickness.—Requirements of Sickness Registration.—Information now Available.—Object Prophylactic as well as Scientific.—Compulsory Notification of Infectious Diseases.—Advantages of Notification.—Methods.—Extension of Notification.—Diseases to be Notified.—Effect on Zymotic Mortality.—National Registration of Infectious Diseases.

THE registration of deaths gives a very imperfect view of the prevalence of disease. Sanitarians would have a greatly increased power of protecting the public health if they could by early information of every case of preventible disease track its development and progress, and adopt measures of prevention. Dr. Lyon Playfair, in 1874, emphasized the importance of registration of sickness in these words: "The record of deaths only registers, as it were, the wrecks which strew the shore, but it gives no account of the vessels which were tossed in the billows of sickness, strained and maimed as they often are by the effects of recurrent storms. Registration of sickness would tell us of the coming storms and enable us to trim our vessels to meet them."

Mortality statistics necessarily "ignore all that precedes the close of life." Can we from them obtain any idea as to the *prevalence of a given disease* in the absence of registration of disease? Under certain circumstances this may be possible, when a disease usually attacks an individual but once in a lifetime, and its fatality has been determined by observation on a sufficiently large scale. Thus in the year 1876 there were 2,297 deaths from scarlet fever in London. In the metropolitan hospitals there were during the same year 1,355 cases, with deaths in a little over 10 per cent. Assuming the same rate of mortality, within and out of the hospitals, there were at least 22,885 cases of scarlet fever in London during that year. But the severer cases were more likely to be taken to the hospital, and the mortality would in that event be greater among hospital patients; on which assumption the total number of scarlet fever patients in London was greater than estimated above. Nearly 70 per cent of the fatal cases occurred among children under five years of age, whence the Registrar-General infers that at least 15,000 out of the 453,171 children living under that age in London, or about 1 in 30, had scarlet fever during the year.

In other cases, however, as rheumatism, ague, asthma, it would be impossible to form even a rough idea of the prevalence of a given disease from its fatality, as it may recur an indefinite number of times in the same individual.

In a few cases, such as hydrophobia, splenic fever, and possibly cancer (which may, however, not recur after operation), the number of deaths may be taken as indicating the number of cases.

It is very fallacious, however, to assume any fixed ratio between sickness and mortality. In order to obtain a rough idea of the prevalence of scarlet fever from the number of deaths and the number treated in hospitals, it was necessary to wait until after the occurrence of a large number of cases, when the information was of no practical value. The *fatality of a given disease varies greatly* in different outbreaks under varying circumstances. The highest ratio of sickness is occasionally found associated with a favourable rate of mortality. Cholera is much less fatal towards the end of an epidemic than at its beginning; so a conclusion drawn simply from the death returns might easily exaggerate the diminution in the prevalence of the disease.

There are some diseases, again, the knowledge of which is desirable, but which do not perceptibly affect the mortality (except in some cases, through secondary consequences), as quinsy, influenza, mumps, chicken-pox, gonorrhœa.

The medical officer of health, who only knows of fatal cases of preventible diseases, often feels himself in the impotent position of a mere recorder of events. If he knew of *every* case, preventive measures could be adopted at an early stage, and the outbreak could be tracked to its true origin, as not a single link in the chain of evidence would be missing.

Death returns are silent about the large mass of common sickness, which, although it may disable a man, is not "unto death." From an economical point of view, this *sickness is more important than deaths*, "for it is the amount and duration of sickness rather than the mortality that tell on the prosperity of a community" (Dr. Dickson). Or as Charles Dickens has stated it: "It concerns a man more to know his risks of the fifty illnesscs that may throw him on his back than the possible date of the one death that must come. We must have a list of killed *and of the wounded too!*"

Local returns of disabling sickness of every description would not only enable us to deal promptly with epidemic disease, but would also throw great light on the influence of season and climate, of social condition, and of trades and manufactures on health, and would thus enable preventive measures of diverse kinds to be brought into action.

It is evident that even were it possible it is hardly required to know of every case of sickness. The lines of demarcation between health and sickness are ill-defined, and the data, particulars of which will be given in a later chapter (page 275), are practically limited to the *disabling diseases*.

Attempts made to Register Sickness.—Without attempting to give a history of the various attempts made in this country to obtain registration of prevalent diseases in different towns, including Dr. B. W. Richardson's experiment, we can only allude to two organized efforts which were for some time successful.

The first was made by the Metropolitan Association of Health officers in 1857, and included sickness of all kinds attended at the

public expense, in hospitals, and by poor law medical officers, dispensaries, workhouses, etc. The returns were contributed voluntarily by the respective medical officers, the general Board of Health undertaking to print and circulate the weekly and quarterly tables. Of 109 hospitals and dispensaries, generally less than 50 contributed; in some cases boards of guardians refused to supply information; and before the expiration of the second year, the tables, which had never been complete for all sickness attended at the public expense, ceased to appear, voluntary co-operation being evidently unequal to the enterprise. It should be noted also that the returns were not entirely trustworthy so far as they went, for the diseases and accidents notified were not all new cases; that many returns represented patients who had come up from country districts for hospital treatment; and that an indefinite number of patients, who wander from hospital to hospital, must have been notified more than once. Dr. Ransome and the Sanitary Association of Manchester and Salford organized in 1860 a system of registration of sickness for these towns which appears to have been very complete and exact, and was not finally abandoned until the compulsory notification of infectious diseases came into force nearly twenty-five years later. An attempt was made, at Dr. Ransome's suggestion, to obtain simultaneously with the returns of disease a record of the mortality occurring amongst the cases reported. This was then compared with the total mortality, and a very fair guess could thus be made as to the total number of cases occurring within the district.

The **Requirements of a Plan** for the registration of disease have been set forth by Dr. Farr as follows, in the supplement to the Registrar-General's Thirty-fifth Annual Report: "The reports of the existing medical officers are of great practical value, and will become more valuable every day. What is wanted is a staff officer in every county or great city, with clerks, to enable him to analyse and publish the results of weekly returns of sickness, to be procured from every district; distinguishing, as the army returns do, the new cases, the recoveries, the deaths reported weekly, and the patients remaining in the several hospitals, dispensaries, and workhouses. These compiled on a uniform plan, when consolidated in the metropolis, would be of national concern. It has been suggested that the returns of sickness should, to save time, be sent to London, and there analysed on a uniform system, as the causes of death are. That with the present postal arrangements is quite practicable. The thing to aim at ultimately is a return of the cases of sickness in the civil population as complete as is now procured from the army in England. It will be an invaluable contribution to therapeutics, as well as to hygiene: for it will enable the therapeutists to determine the duration and the fatality of all forms of disease, under the several existing systems of treatment, in the various sanitary and social conditions of the people. Illusion will be dispelled, quackery, as completely as astrology, suppressed, a science of therapeutics created, suffering diminished, life shielded from many dangers. The national returns of cases and of causes of death will be an arsenal which the genius of English healers cannot fail to turn to account."

Information now Available.—1. Under an order made by the Local Government Board in February, 1879, it is incumbent on all district and workhouse medical officers appointed since that date to furnish the medical officers of health with returns of pauper sickness and deaths, as well as to notify the outbreak of dangerous infectious disease. A similar obligation has been imposed upon medical officers of district schools appointed after June, 1879.

By means of these returns of pauper sickness a fair estimate of the prevalence of disease among the poorest classes can be obtained. The information is not quite so valuable as might be expected, especially in large towns, owing to the fact that only a small proportion of cases of enteric fever, diphtheria, etc., are treated at the patients' own home; the chief exception to this rule being diarrhœa.

2. The keeper of a common lodging house is bound to give information to the local authority of any case of dangerous infectious disease occurring on his premises.

3. Where bye-laws are in force in any district in relation to houses occupied by more than one family, the householder may be compelled to notify the occurrence of infectious disease to the local authority.

4. In addition to these sources of compulsory information, information is usually available from medical men where disinfection or removal of patients is required, from the clergy, from school-board officers, and from the post-office authorities when any of their employés suffer from infectious illness.

If the information accumulated by Friendly Societies were available, it would possess great value; and a combination of information from this source, and from other sick clubs, from medical charities, and from the poor law guardians, would supply a fairly good system of registration of illness for each district. None of these would, however, suffice for sanitary purposes; they would not furnish the necessary information in regard to such children's diseases as measles and whooping cough, and but imperfect information as to scarlet fever. For these and like diseases compulsory notification of infectious diseases is essential.

What may be regarded as an ideal system is that in force in the army and navy, where every case of sickness is tabulated as to character, duration, and result. Although it is not likely that any such complete returns will be obtained for the civil population, it may be hoped that in the not very distant future compulsory notification will not be confined to infectious diseases.

Compulsory Notification of Infectious Diseases.—The main object of registration of sickness is prophylactic, and from this standpoint the registration of infectious diseases is supremely important. Such registration, in order to be of value, must be *compulsory*. Whenever it has been simply voluntary and optional, the returns have been invariably imperfect and incomplete. Voluntary notification has been tried in a few places, medical men being paid a fee for every case information of which they furnish to the sanitary authority. The result has been only very partial. The medical practitioner is by possibility subjected to odium and accused of a breach of professional secrecy when he notifies, unless the notification is compulsory. Such partial information is not trustworthy as indicating the prevalence of a disease, though it is better than none; nor is it efficacious in stopping the spread of disease. The more cases the medical officer of health knows of and the wider the basis on which his etiological deductions can be built, the more likely are preventive measures to be successful. It must not be supposed, however, that compulsory notification of infectious diseases forms a complete means of meeting and combating infectious diseases. "We do not only seek to suppress them when they arise, but to prevent their origin" (Ransome); and to this end, we require to study thoroughly their natural history, their habitats, and the conditions under which they develop and recur.

Advantages of Notification.—1. Early prophylactic measures can be taken, and thus it may be possible to choke epidemics at their birth. The centres of infection are diminished not only by the isolation of those actually ill, but also by preventing the commingling of "suspects," who have been exposed to infection, with others. In the case of small-pox, early notification allows time for successful vaccination of exposed persons. More effective isolation in hospital of persons without proper home isolation can be enforced. Dr. Tatham reports in regard to Salford, that in 1883, the first year of work under its local notification Act, only 26 per cent of the cases notified were removed to the hospital, while during 1887-8, the proportion had reached nearly 50 per cent. The work of disinfection is very largely increased whenever notification is adopted.

2. The attendance at school of children from the infected family can be controlled.

3. Incidentally the inspection made leads to the discovery of other conditions likely to spread disease; as, for instance, milk supply, business of laundry, tailor, etc.

4. A vast amount of inspection of bad premises follows on the information received, and sanitary measures are adopted.

5. The necessary inspections have a marked educational influence on parents, householders, teachers, etc.; and lead to increased care in taking measures to prevent the spread of infection.

Methods of Notification.—The different systems of compulsory notification in force are: (1) notification compulsory only on the householder; (2) compulsory only on the medical attendant; (3) compulsory on both separately; (4) compulsory on the doctor to certify to the householder, and on the latter to notify to the local authority or the medical officer of health. Of the fifty-two towns in which compulsory notification prevails, in all but two (Aberdeen and Edinburgh) the occupier is bound to give notice to the local authority in case no medical man is in attendance. In nine towns the householder is exempt from notification if a doctor is in attendance (Ashton-under-Lyne, Dewsbury, Hartlepool, Manchester, Norwich, Preston, Rotherham, Edinburgh, Aberdeen). At only one town (Greenock) is the doctor exempt from a share in the notification. In Bradford, Norwich, and Nottingham it is compulsory on the medical attendant to furnish a certificate of the disease to the householder, and the latter is responsible for its transmission to the local authority. This method seems clumsy and roundabout; but in practice it works well, and relieves the practitioner from any possible odium connected with the divulgence of his patient's complaint. It puts the real onus on the guardians of the patient, who are the only persons who owe this duty to the State.

Notification, to be of service, should be early and complete, and notification by the householder is probably insufficient for this purpose. It has failed at Greenock. Even where notification is compulsory on the householder, in practice information is nearly always given by the medical attendant; by being associated in compulsion with the householder he avoids any possible odium; and it is probable that this "dual method" will be the one approved by the Local Government Board, and recommended for universal adoption. It is urged that this method will, in the event of secrecy being desired, prevent a medical man being called in; but the same thing would on this supposition happen if the onus of notification rested solely on the householder. For the doctor would be bound to give evidence that the nature of the illness had been stated by him to the householder, and the latter would in consequence have no excuse for not notifying.

When notification has been in force for some time, the theoretical difficulties have been found to dwindle, and there is usually little or no friction. The *difficulties urged* are as follows: (1) the desire of the doctor to respect his patient's confidence; and, in connection with this, (2) the desire to avoid publicity. There is, however, not the slightest need that the returns should cease to be strictly confidential; and the public interests may be guarded with full regard to the welfare of the sick and non-interference with trade and other concerns. (3) There is the difficulty of hospital accommodation. To secure the full benefits of notification, hospital accommodation must be provided, and where necessary there must be power of compulsory removal. (4) In towns where the medical officer of health is in practice medical men object to give information concerning their private cases. With tact on the part of the medical officer, this difficulty can be overcome; but the best arrangement is for the medical officer to have charge of a sufficiently large area to justify his not engaging in private practice.

Extension of Notification.—As the law stands at present, it rests with individual towns to apply for the necessary powers. Three towns, Bury, Manchester, and Salford, obtained provisional orders from the Local Government Board, which were subsequently confirmed by Parliament. Most corporations who have obtained this compulsory power have preferred the more expensive machinery of a local Act.

The Local Government Board has within the last year (December, 1887) sent round a circular to each notification town, asking for particulars of the working of the system; and it may be hoped that the time is now ripe for an Imperial measure on the subject for the whole country. The principle of notification is already fully acknowledged by the Legislature in the case of towns where byelaws are in force for houses let in lodgings, and in regard to common lodging houses. Such piecemeal and class legislation should be extended to the whole community. It would appear also that more thought is taken by the Legislature for cattle than for human beings; for by the Contagious Diseases (Animals) Act, of 1878, every cattle owner is required under heavy penalties to report without delay any outbreak of infectious disease among his stock to the local authority.

Diseases to be Notified. — Small-pox, Scarlet Fever, Diphtheria, Typhus Fever, and Typhoid Fever, are usually the only diseases included in the schedule of notifiable diseases. In a few towns Measles is notified; and considering how great mortality this disease may cause, there is strong reason for including it in every instance. Epidemic Diarrhœa does not appear to be notified in any town, though we think there are very strong reasons for its addition to the list.

Effect of Notification on Zymotic Mortality.—An attempt has been recently made to determine by appeal to figures whether compulsory notification diminishes the prevalence and fatality of infectious diseases. We doubt whether such an appeal to figures can be trusted, because it is hardly possible that the periods compared should fulfil an indispensable condition when comparisons are instituted; viz., that *other things shall be equal.* There are collateral sources of error. Notification often is not the only improvement which has occurred in notification towns. Alongside of notification various sanitary measures may have been taken, tending to a diminution of infectious disease. At the same time it must be remembered that after such a disease as measles or scarlet fever has gone through a town it exhausts the supply of persons prone to these diseases; and apart altogether from any sanitary measures, some years must elapse before sufficient material has accumulated to furnish fuel for another outbreak. In addition to this, there are probably periodic cyclical influences, the nature of which is imperfectly known, but which have important bearings on the prevalence of a given disease. So that neither on the one hand, the comparative absence of a given infectious disease since notification came into force, nor, on the other hand, its increased prevalence, proves the utility or inutility of notification.

The question is mixed up also with that of hospital accommodation and isolation. Notification is but a means to an end. There may be no good results from it if the patients notified cannot be properly isolated.

It should be remembered also that the materials available for drawing conclusions are very scanty, and that in many of the notification towns the period since notification began is too short to enable valid conclusions to be drawn. Perhaps the best example of the value of notification, combined with a good sanitary organization, is that of Leicester, cited by Dr. Seaton. During the six years preceding 1887, in London, without any compulsory notification, the average annual mortality from small-pox was 26 per 100,000, while in Leicester it was only 1 per 100,000, spite of the large proportion of unvaccinated children.

Dr. Tatham, Medical Officer of Health for Salford, has collected the statistics of the five following diseases from 41 towns, representing a population of over 4 millions, in which notification is in force; and from his Annual Report (Salford, 1887) we abstract the appended table.

Rate of Sickness per 100,000 of Population in 41 towns from the several Infectious Diseases, notification of which is compulsory under the Local Acts of Parliament.

	1883.	1884.	1885.	1886.	1887.
Small Pox . .	20	12	19	10	8
Scarlet Fever .	359	381	364	412	690
Diphtheria . .	33	39	26	33	46
Typhus Fever .	14	10	11	9	7
Enteric Fever .	121	155	134	140	129

While, however, deprecating a premature appeal to statistics in a problem where the conditions necessarily vary so widely, we must state our earnest conviction that universal notification of infectious disease, combined with the strictest isolation in hospitals or elsewhere, constitutes an immensely beneficial sanitary measure, the importance of which can scarcely be exaggerated.

National Registration of Infectious Diseases.—In a paper read at the meeting of the British Medical Association in August, 1888, Dr. Tatham drew attention to this subject, which is complementary to that of local compulsory notification, and if carried out would probably be of almost equal value to the public health. Although there are already 52 notification towns, no machinery is available for making the local information generally serviceable. Seeing this defect, Dr. Tatham, at the beginning of 1888, made a private arrangement with the medical officers of health of 32 other notification towns, by which he should receive from them weekly returns of the cases notified in each town. These were tabulated by him, and then circulated confidentially amongst the contributing medical officers early in the succeeding week. The practicability of this plan having been fully established, Dr. Tatham brought the matter to the attention of the Local Government Board, in the hope that they would take it over as a "going concern." There can be no doubt that they are the proper authority, whose duty it should be to publish these returns. Many of the local authorities, on the strength of the representations of their medical officers, petitioned the Local Government Board to take the matter in hand. The Board then addressed a circular of inquiry to the local authorities, whether in the event of the Board undertaking the publication of weekly returns of sickness, the individual authorities would agree to furnish the Board with the requisite local returns. Favourable answers were generally given to this circular; but no further steps have hitherto been taken (December, 1888).

Such a system would form the natural complement of local notification of infectious diseases. It would enable every medical officer to know what infectious diseases were prevalent in neighbouring towns, to watch their progress, and take precautionary measures against the invasion of his own area. To be forewarned is to be forearmed.

While these pages are passing through the press (Feb., 1889), the medical journals announce that the Local Government Board has just undertaken the tabulation and distribution of the statistics of cases of sickness notified to the sanitary authorities of those towns in which the notification of infectious disease is compulsory. Only the co-operating towns receive the table summarising the statistics of these notification towns; and it is marked "not for publication." We may reasonably expect that this experiment will end in a national registration of infectious disease, and similar tabulation and distribution of the national statistics by the Local Government Board.

CHAPTER IV.

MARRIAGES.

Methods of Estimating Marriages.—Causes of High Marriage-Rate in Towns.—Influence of National Prosperity on Marriage-Rate.—General Decline in Marriage-Rate.—Marriage Calendar.—Marriages and Re-marriages.—Ages at Marriage.—Occupation as Influencing Age at Marriage.—Marriage of Minors.—Duration of Married Life.—Fecundity of Marriage.—Relation between Marriage and Population.—Proportion of Population Unmarried.—Signatures in Marriage Register.

MARRIAGE statistics possess great interest for all who are concerned with the welfare of the people, affording as they do a valuable index of national prosperity, and incidentally throwing an interesting light on the progress of elementary education.

Estimation of Marriages.—1. The usual method is to state the proportion to the actual population, or the number per 1,000 living. Although this method is fairly reliable in comparing the same town or community in successive years, it might lead to some inaccuracy if employed in comparing different communities in the same year; inasmuch as, owing to varying age and sex constitution, the number of marriageable persons, living in different communities, must vary considerably. It is, however, the only method at present available in comparing different communities, and is the one adopted in the following table:—

Marriage-Rate per 1,000 *of Population in*

Years.	England and Wales.	Scotland.	Ireland.	France.	German Empire.	Austria.	Italy.	Norway.	Denmark.
1871	16·7	14·3	10·7	14·4	—	18·9	14·9	13·3	14·6
1872	17·4	15·1	10·0	19·5	20·6	18·6	15·0	14·0	15·0
1873	17·6	15·5	9·6	17·7	20·0	18·8	15·9	14·5	16·2
1874	17·0	15·2	9·2	16·6	19·1	18·1	15·3	15·3	16·4
1875	16·7	14·8	9·1	16·4	18·2	17·1	16·8	15·7	17·0
1876	16·5	15·0	9·9	15·8	17·0	16·5	16·3	15·4	17·1
1877	15·7	14·4	9·3	15·1	16·0	15·0	15·4	15·1	16·1
1878	15·2	13·4	9·5	15·1	15·4	15·2	14·2	14·6	14·8
1879	14·4	12·8	8·7	15·1	15·0	15·5	15·0	13·5	14·7
1880	14·9	13·2	7·8	14·9	15·0	15·2	13·8	13·3	15·2
1881	15·1	13·9	8·5	15·0	14·9	16·0	16·2	12·8	15·6
1882	15·5	14·1	8·6	14·8	15·4	16·4	15·7	13·4	15·4
1883	15·4	14·0	8·5	15·0	15·4	15·7	16·0	13·2	15·4
1884	15·0	13·5	9·1	15·3	15·7	15·7	16·4	13·7	15·6
1885	14·4	12·9	8·6	14·9	15·8	15·2	15·8	13·3	15·1
1886	14·1	12·4	8·4	14·8	15·8	15·5	15·6	13·1	14·2
1887	14·2	12·5	8·7	14·6	15·6	15·6	16·5	—	14·0

2. The more accurate method of estimating the marriage-rate for comparative purposes is to base it on the enumerated or estimated number of bachelors, spinsters, widowers, and widows living at marriageable ages. The number of these can be obtained for the census year from the census returns for each county and every urban sanitary district with a population of over 50,000 persons; and as there is every reason to believe that the proportion does not vary appreciably from year to year, the same method of estimation for increase of this portion of the population can be adopted as described (p. 6) for the whole population.

The marriage-rate, as estimated by the ordinary method, is fairly trustworthy for successive years for the same country. As shown in the preceding table, it was very low in 1886, and in fact was the lowest since civil registration began. The highest had been 17·9 in 1853; the next highest 17·6 in 1873, as compared with 14·4 in 1885 and 14·1 in 1886.

Higher Marriage-Rate in Towns.—The marriage-rate is

always higher in large towns than in rural districts. This is chiefly explained by the fact that a large number of young country-people resort to populous districts, where, owing to the presence of large trades and manufactures, higher wages can be secured, and there they marry. In towns there is nearly always an excess of persons between twenty and forty years of age. Many also resort to towns merely to be married, subsequently returning to rural districts.

Influence of National Prosperity on Marriage-Rate.—Dr. Farr has described the marriage-rate as the barometer of prosperity (present in part, but future anticipated prosperity in still greater part), just as the funds are the barometer of credit. So we find that the marriages of England increase as "the result of peace after war, abundance after dearth, high wages after want of employment, speculation after languid enterprise, confidence after distrust, national triumphs after national disasters."

The same conclusion is borne out by the fact, frequently alluded to by the Registrar-General in his reports, that the marriage-rate varies in the same direction as the value of British exports, the average price of wheat, and the amount per head of population cleared out at the Bankers' Clearing House. The coincidence, it should be pointed out, is one in direction, but not in degree. Twice only in twenty-two years did the marriage-rate and exports move in different directions, while the marriage-rate and imports moved diversely seven times in twenty-two years.

The fact that marriages increase as the price of wheat rises is explained by the Registrar-General as follows: Evidently the price of wheat, and therefore of food, has ceased to be the one determining factor rendering marriage justifiable or the reverse. The amount of wages is more important than the price of food, and the wages are determined by the demand for labour, and this, speaking generally, by the amount and value of the goods produced and exported. Consequently the marriage-rate fluctuates with the exports of British goods rather than with the cheapness of food; and this explains the fact that marriages do not increase when food is cheap. It does not explain, however, their increase when food is dear; and the Registrar-General (48th Annual Report) suggests that with increased wages, or an increased number of persons earning wages, there is a greater consumption of bread and a consequent rise in the price of wheat. He acknowledges, however, that the question requires the attention of experts, and a portion of his reasoning is certainly undermined by the fact, for which we can vouch, that in agricultural districts, like Lincolnshire, it is the price of wheat which determines the amount of wages, and not *vice versâ*.

General Decline in Marriage-Rate.—The preceding table shows that in this country there has been a considerable and almost continuous fall in the number of marriages, which set in with 1874. A similar decline is shown in other States; in France, Prussia, and the German Empire it set in a year earlier. In the latter countries the diminution appears greater, owing to the abnormally high marriage-rate in 1872, at the conclusion of the Franco-Prussian war. It is evident that, as the decline in the marriage-rate is not confined to England, it cannot be regarded as indicating any falling off in the prosperity of this country, as compared with other parts of Europe.

Marriage Calendar.—The Registrar-General's statistics show that most marriages occur in December, October, April, and June. The greater number of marriages in December, April, and June are accounted for by the festive periods of Christmas, Easter, and Whitsuntide coinciding with these months; while October is the period after the harvest, when the agricultural labourer has comparative leisure as well as money in his pocket. The month of May, for some unknown reason, is lowest on the list as regards number of marriages. The favourite days in the week for marriages are Saturday, Monday, and Sunday.

Marriages and Remarriages.—In the year 1886, of the total marriages 87·6 per cent. were of bachelors and 12·4 per cent. of widowers. Of the bachelors who married (171,664 in number), 95·6 per cent. married spinsters and 4·4 per cent.

widows. Of the widowers who remarried (24,407 in number), 62 per cent. married spinsters and 38 per cent. widows. Of the women married during the same year, 91·4 per cent. were spinsters and 8·6 per cent. widows. Of the spinsters (179,301 in number), 91·6 per cent. were married to bachelors and 8·4 per cent. to widowers. Of the 16,770 widows who were re-married during the year, 44·7 per cent. were married to bachelors and 55·3 per cent. to widowers.

Ages at Marriage.—The statistics under this head are imperfect, owing to the phrases "full age," "minor," "under age," being frequently inserted in the register. There is evidence, however, of steady improvement in this respect; for while in 1851 in 63 per cent. of the total marriages the precise age was not stated, in 1861 the proportion had fallen to 37, in 1871 to 29, in 1885 to 8·5, and in 1886 to 6·9 per cent. It is unfortunate that such statement of age at marriage is not compulsory, as it would form an important datum in determining the relative fecundity of different populations.

Of the 93·1 per cent. of the total marriages in 1886 in which the age of the contracting parties was stated, the mean age of the women married was 25·9 years, and of the men 28·2 years. Taking marriages and remarriages separately, the mean age of widowers married was 43·8 years; of widows, 40·1 years; of bachelors, 26·2; and of spinsters, 24·6 years. Postponement of marriage of course limits the childbearing period; and a portion of the lowering of birth-rate which has occurred of late years may be ascribed to this cause.

Age at Marriage (in Years) of

Year.	Bachelors.	Spinsters.
1880	25·8	24·4
1881	25·9	24·4
1882	25·9	24·4
1883	25·9	24·4
1884	26·0	24·5
1885	26·1	24·6
1886	26·2	24·6
1887	26·2	24·7

The mean age at marriage has been gradually rising since 1873. In that year there was great prosperity, and the marriage-rate was at its maximum, the mean age of bachelors at marriage being 25·6, and of spinsters 24·2 years, the lowest recorded. Since then the mean age at marriage has gradually risen, the figures for 1887 (see above table) being the highest yet recorded. It appears, therefore, that when the marriages are few in number, they are also delayed to a somewhat later period of life.

Mr. C. Ansell in his "Statistics of Families in the Upper and Professional Classes" (page 44), found that the mean age at marriage of bachelors of these classes during the period 1840 to 1871 was 29·95 years.

The following table from the Registrar-General's Annual Report for 1886 gives the relative age at marriage in different social conditions, widows and widowers being left out of account.

Average Ages at Marriage of Bachelors and Spinsters in Occupational Groups, 1884–1885.

Occupations.	Bachelors.	Spinsters.	Difference between Ages of Husband and Wife.
Miners	24·06	22·46	— 1·60
Textile hands	24·38	23·43	— 0·95
Shoemakers, Tailors	24·92	24·31	— 0·61
Artisans	25·35	23·70	— 1·65
Labourers	25·56	23 66	— 1·90
Commercial Clerks	26·25	24·43	— 1·82
Shopkeepers, Shopmen	26·67	24 22	— 2·45
Farmers and Sons	29·23	26 91	— 2·32
Professional and Independent Class	31·22	26·40	— 4·82

It will be seen from this table that in the groups in which men marry early, so do the women. Thus in the case of miners and textile hands the mean age at marriage in both men and women is at its lowest; while in farmers and those of the professional and independent classes there is the highest mean age at marriage of both. It will be observed also that the more advanced the mean age, the greater becomes the difference between the age of husband and wife.

Marriage of Minors.—Spite of the gradually rising mean age at marriage, the marriages of minors do not show any corresponding decrease. 8·1 per cent. of the bachelors (13,079) and 23·6 per cent. of the spinsters (39,533) whose ages at marriage were stated in 1886 were under 21 years of age; and in 6·2 per cent. of the marriages between bachelors and spinsters whose ages were stated *both* contracting parties were minors.

The following table shows, without discrimination between first marriages and re-marriages, the proportion of marriages per 1,000 total marriages which occurred in successive years under 21 years of age:—

Proportion per 1,000 *Marriages, occurring under* 21 *years of age.*

Years.	Men.	Women.
1841	44	133
1846	43	137
1851	50	157
1856	57	183
1861	64	195
1866	67	200
1871	79	220
1876	83	220
1881	72	214
1882	76	220
1883	74	218
1884	73	213
1885	70	210
1886	67	206
1887	65	202

To ascertain more exactly the proportion of women marrying under age, we should require to know accurately the number of unmarried men and women living under 21 years of age. Dr. Farr, acting on this method (35th Annual Report), came to the conclusion, from figures given in the following table, that there was an increasing tendency to early marriage among the young people of this country, though since 1872 the proportion of marriages under age as thus measured has probably decreased (see table, page 49).

Number of Marriages per 1,000 *persons living under* 21.

Years.	Men.	Women.
1850–52	7·6	24·3
1860–62	9·5	29·6
1870–72	11·8	34·1

Fecundity of Marriage.—Marriage being the great institution by which the population is chiefly regulated, it becomes necessary to consider the conditions regulating the fertility of marriage. The two most important of these are the duration of married life, and the age at which marriage is contracted by women.

Dr. Farr in his census report for 1871 stated that 8 out of every 10 brides and bridegrooms at their first marriage are between 20 and 30 years of age, the mean of both sexes at their first marriage being 25, that of the bridegroom 25·65 years, and of the bride 24·3 years. The mean time that a couple of such lives survive is, as shown by calculations, 27 years, which represents the duration of married life, and approximately the time during which the issue of the marriage enjoy the joint protection of both parents. The further mean lifetime of the surviving parent is in the case of the father 9·44 years, of the mother 11·31 years.

Late marriages, by shortening the probable duration of married life, increase the proportional number of orphans.

The *age at marriage* is the chief factor controlling the proportion of children to a marriage, the age of the wife being the most important element, because of the fact that child-bearing is limited practically between the 16th and 45th years of life. The fathers and mothers of nearly half the children born are, according to Dr. Farr, under 30 years of age. If all the women at 30 should marry, and none before, the births would be reduced to about two-thirds of their present number; and if the marriage age were postponed to 35, the births would fall to one-third of their present number, and the population would rapidly decline. For not only (*a*) would the number of births in each generation diminish, but also (*b*) the interval between the births of successive generations would lengthen, the length of life remaining the same according to the hypothesis.

It has been doubted whether early marriages are really more fruitful than later ones; and this is certain, that women who have married at about 17 or 18 frequently cease child-bearing before they are 30, the reproductive powers being exhausted. But even supposing the fertility of early and late marriages to be identical, the number of children in the latter is less because of (*a*) the greater length of the generation, and (*b*) the fact that many who would have been parents have died before reaching the later age of marriage.

The following table, from the Registrar-General's 40th Annual Report, gives the comparative fecundity of various European States. During the three years 1876–79 the average number of births to a marriage in England was 4·57.

Comparative Fecundity in Different European States.

Years.	European States.	Births to a Marriage.
1876	Italy	5·15
,,	Prussia	4·92
,,	Sweden	4·84
,,	Netherlands. . .	4·83
,,	England	4·63
,,	Belgium	4·48
1870	Spain	4·47
1876	Denmark . . .	4·24
,,	Austria	3·73
,,	France	3·42

Assuming that the interval between the mean age of marriage and the mean age of mothers in England is six years, then the legitimate births in 1874, divided by the average number of marriages in the three years 1867–9, will give the average number of births to a marriage, which was 4·57. In 1864 it was 4·30, but the apparent increase is probably owing to improved registration of births.

According to the last census in France, 20 per cent. of the families in that country have no children, 24 per cent. have one child, 22 per cent. 2 children, 15 per cent. 3 children, 9 per cent. 4 children, 5 per cent. 5 children, 3 per cent. 6 children, and 2 per cent. have 7 or more children; while there are on an average 259 children to 100 fertile marriages.

Proportion of Population Unmarried.—The census report of 1851 shows that of the population at ages of 20 and upwards, about 1 in 10 men and 1 in 8 women may be referred to the category of those never marrying. It is evident, therefore, that celibacy as well as marriage without children is the natural state of a portion of the population.

The relative number of married and unmarried women during the decennium 1851–60 is shown in the following table:

Married and Unmarried Women aged 15–55 *in Years* 1851–60.

	Number in Each Class.		Percentage in Each Class.	
	England.	Scotland.	England.	Scotland.
Women . .	5,437,769	867,062	100·00	100·00
Wives . . .	2,843,374	383,271	52·29	44·20
Spinsters and Widows. .	2,594,395	483,791	47·71	55·80

Thus in England 52 in 100 women of the age 15–55 were wives, while in Scotland only 44 were such.

The following table, arranged by Dr. Longstaff from the 1881 census report, gives the numbers and conjugal condition of both sexes at the last census:—

Excess of Males or Females at Different Groups of Ages, together with their Conjugal Condition.

Ages and Condition.	Males.		Females.	
	Numbers.	Excess over Females.	Numbers.	Excess over Males.
Children under 15 .	4,728,466	—	4,740,125	11,659
Unmarried, 15–35 .	2,704,062	72,629	2,631,433	—
,, 35–45 .	195,427	—	233,820	38,393
,, 45– .	200,255	—	292,151	91,896
Married, 15–35 . .	1,469,040	—	1,778,237	309,197
,, 35– . .	2,907,858	248,133	2,659,725	—
Widowed, all ages .	434,794	—	999,046	564,252
Total . . .	12,639,902	320,762	13,334,537	1,015,397
Balance, Excess of Females . . .	—	694,635	—	—

Signatures in Marriage Register.—These throw an interesting sidelight on the state of elementary education in this country, as indicated by the ability to sign the marriage register.

Proportion Unable to sign Marriage Register.

Year.	1841.	1851.	1861.	1871.	1881.	1887.
Out of 1,000 Men Married, No. unable to sign Register	326	308	246	194	135	91
Out of 1,000 Women Married, No. unable to sign Register	488	453	347	268	177	106
Out of 1,000 Persons Married, both unable to sign Register	?	225	161	113	64	34

In the country as a whole, the number of men unable to write is considerably less than of women, though the difference between the two sexes, as shown in the above table, is rapidly diminishing. Taking the counties separately there is great discrepancy, the general rule being, according to the Registrar-General, that in agricultural counties the male, and in mining and industrial counties the female, is the worse educated sex.

CHAPTER V.

BIRTHS.

Estimation of Birth-rate.—History of Registration of Births.—Birth statistics of Counties of England and Wales.—Influence of Social Position and National Prosperity.—Influence of Nationality.—Still-Births.—Proportion of Males and Females at Birth.—Illegitimacy.—Influence of Early Marriage and of Education on Illegitimacy.—The Malthusian hypothesis.—Laws of Increase of Population and of Subsistence.—Influence of Birth-rate on Age-Constitution of Population.—Natural Increase of Population.

THE consideration in the last chapter of marriages and their average fecundity naturally opens the way to a discussion of birth statistics. Such statistics are of value in giving information as to the rate of increase of the population, and the age and sex-distribution of the population, in addition to their great social interest, especially when the statistics of illegitimacy are included.

Estimation of Birth-rate.—The birth-rate may be estimated by the following plans, of which the second is the more accurate, though not so easily available for ordinary purposes. (1) It is reckoned as a rate per 1,000 of the population living at all ages, in the middle of the year. This may be described as a *crude birth-rate.* It is satisfactory when used for the same community in a series of years, or in comparing the birth-rates of communities whose populations are known to be nearly if not quite identical in their age and sex-composition. If, however, the number living at child-bearing years differs in two populations, the birth-rate per 1,000 of the total population would vary from this cause, apart altogether from varying fecundity of the two populations. Thus in 1870 the number of persons in the United States aged 20–60 years amounted to 43·9 per cent. of the total population; while in France the corresponding number was 53·7 per cent.

When more accuracy is required, we must (2) calculate the proportion the births registered bear to the women living at child-bearing years; *i.e.*, roughly between about 16 and 45 years. These are shown by the census returns for each urban and rural sanitary district; and as the age and sex composition, except in very abnormal cases, does not vary materially in an intercensal period, the same proportion of women aged 16–45 to the total population holds good throughout the intervening period between any two census enumerations. A birth-rate obtained in this way is doubtless more accurate in comparing one country with another, and even different towns or districts of the same country; but the crude birth-rate is sufficiently reliable for ordinary purposes.

(3) It has been proposed to estimate the fecundity of a population by determining the proportion of births to each marriage. This method, however, makes no allowance for illegitimate births.

To ascertain the number of births to each marriage, the annual births should be divided by the annual marriages of some previous year. It is assumed that the interval between the average age at marriage and at the birth of children is six years; and on this assumption in the table on page 51 the legitimate births in 1876 are divided by the marriages registered six years earlier.

Defects in Registration of Births.—Prior to the operation of the Civil Registration Act of 1837, there were no trustworthy birth statistics. In the earlier years of the operation of the Act the birth registration was undoubtedly deficient, Dr. Farr estimating the deficiency during the $39\frac{1}{2}$ years ending with 1876 at 5 per cent. The registration of births was first made compulsory by the Births and Deaths Registration Act of 1874; and it is probable that at the present time the failure of registration is very small, and chiefly confined to illegitimate births. There are two grave defects in the Birth Registers of the United Kingdom. The ages of the mothers at the birth of each of their children are not stated, nor is the order of their birth recorded, so that the number of children borne by women at different ages, and the total number in the course of their lives, cannot be ascertained in this country.

Births Statistics of England and Wales.

Years.	Births to 1,000 Living.			Illegitimate Births in 1,000 Births.	Births of Males to 1,000 Births of Females.
	Total.	Legitimate.	Illegitimate.		
1841-50	32·6	30·5	2·1	67	1049
1851–60	34·1	31·9	2·2	65	1046
1861–70	35·2	33·1	2·1	61	1042
1871–75	35·5	33·7	1·8	52	1039
1876	36·3	34·6	1·7	47	1038
1877	36·0	34·3	1·7	47	1036
1878	35·6	33·9	1·7	47	1042
1879	34·7	33·0	1·7	48	1036
1880	34·2	32·6	1·6	48	1036
1881	33·9	32·2	1·7	49	1039
1882	33·7	32·1	1·6	49	1038
1883	33·3	31·7	1·6	48	1035
1884	33·3	31·7	1·6	47	1041
1885	32·5	30·9	1·5	48	1040
1886	32·4	30·9	1·5	47	1038
1887	31·4	29·9	1·5	48	1039

It will be seen from the above table that the birth-rate in this country is steadily decreasing, the comparatively low figures in the earlier years of the preceding table being at least in part ascribable to imperfect registration.

The birth-rate varies considerably under different circumstances. Some of these will be now considered. The variation in different **counties** is shown by the table on pages 58 and 59 from the Registrar-General's 49th Annual Report.

The lowest rates occur in the agricultural, and the highest in mining and industrial districts. Thus, in the table referred to, we find the birth-rate in Staffordshire 36·1, in Durham 36·2, in Lancashire 33·7, as compared with 29·8 in Dorsetshire, 29·5 in Devonshire, and 27·3 in Herefordshire.

The higher birth-rate in **urban populations**, which are to a great extent included in mining and industrial districts, is owing in part to the higher marriage-rate, and in part to the earlier marriage of women, and the greater mortality among infants, which, by shortening the period of suckling, diminishes the intervals of child-bearing. But the chief reason is doubtless the fact that in urban populations there is a greater proportion of women at child-bearing ages.

Social Position has a considerable influence on the birth-rate, though there are very few data to determine this point. The fallacy involved in the fact that people's social position tends to improve as their ages advance should be remembered. We have already seen (page 48) that persons of the higher classes marry at a later age than others. There are serious fallacies involved in comparing the crude birth-rate of two populations. Thus Mr. Chadwick compared the metropolitan births, which at the time of his remarks were 1 in 37 of the population, with those of Herefordshire, which were 1 in 44; but Mr. Neison showed that this difference was largely explained by the fact that while the population aged 20 to 40 was 36·33 per cent. of the total population in London, it was only 28·39 per cent in Herefordshire.

The influence of **National Prosperity** on the birth-rate is in the same direction as its influence on the marriage-rate (page 45). A high birth-rate is due to prosperity, unless artificial and voluntary checks to population are introduced. The numbers of the population are increased by an abundance of the necessaries of life, and reduced by converse influences, as famine, epidemics, and other calamities. The only exception to the rule that national prosperity is accompanied by a high birth-rate occurs when, from any cause, early and improvident marriages or illegitimate births increase to a large extent.

REGISTRATION COUNTY.	Births to 1,000 Living.		Illegitimate Births to 1,000 Births.		Males Born to 1,000 Females Born.		Deaths to 1,000 Living.				Deaths of Children under one Year to 1,000 Births.	
	Ten Years 1876–85.	1886.	Ten Years 1876–85.	1886.	Ten Years 1876–85.	1886.	Ten Years 1876-85. Persons.	1886. Persons.	1886. Males.	1886. Females.	Ten Years 1876–85.	1886.
ENGLAND	34·4	32·4	48	47	1038	1038	20·1	19·3	20·3	18·3	142	149
I.—LONDON	34·7	32·4	39	38	1039	1041	21·4	19·9	21·6	18·4	152	159
II.—SOUTH EASTERN.												
Surrey (*extra-metropolitan*)	30·5	28·7	39	41	1033	1016	16·3	16·0	17·3	14·8	112	120
Kent (*extra-metropolitan*)	32·2	31·7	43	43	1044	1028	17·4	17·8	18·5	17·1	118	130
Sussex	29·7	27·4	51	52	1045	1035	16·4	16·1	17·2	15·0	110	121
Hampshire	31·2	31·4	44	41	1036	1022	17·8	19·3	20·4	18·2	112	131
Berkshire	31·2	29·9	48	51	1041	1036	17·3	17·0	17·8	16·1	110	121
III.—SOUTH MIDLAND.												
Middlesex (*extra-metrop.*)	33·2	35·1	35	32	1041	1041	17·5	17·8	19·2	16·5	128	142
Hertfordshire	31·1	30·3	55	54	1035	1072	17·5	18·2	19·0	17·4	112	115
Buckinghamshire	32·2	32·4	53	46	1043	1026	17·9	18·5	19·0	18·1	122	132
Oxfordshire	31·0	30·8	56	57	1037	1094	17·7	18·2	19·3	17·1	117	121
Northamptonshire	33·9	32·1	45	45	1040	1032	18·3	18·3	18·9	17·7	135	143
Huntingdonshire	29·6	29·7	49	46	1054	980	17·2	19·3	20·5	18·2	114	111
Bedfordshire	32·5	33·2	68	64	1027	1079	18·7	18·9	20·6	17·4	138	137
Cambridgeshire	30·9	30·1	55	54	1043	1045	17·9	19·5	20·3	18·8	128	140
IV.—EASTERN.												
Essex	34·5	36·8	36	34	1034	1058	18·0	19·0	19·7	18·2	125	134
Suffolk	32·0	32·2	58	59	1036	1015	18·2	18·7	19·7	17·8	118	132
Norfolk	31·2	31·8	77	72	1046	1068	19·0	19·4	20·8	18·1	139	149
V.—SOUTH WESTERN.												
Wiltshire	30·8	29·4	48	48	1033	1012	17·9	17·5	18·0	17·0	105	108
Dorsetshire	29·3	29·8	50	46	1037	1029	16·9	17·6	18·1	17·1	102	105
Devonshire	29·6	29·5	48	46	1037	1055	19·0	19·7	20·7	18·9	121	126
Cornwall	29·4	30·6	63	60	1051	1109	19·9	22·1	23·1	21·3	138	160
Somersetshire	30·6	30·1	44	42	1041	1048	18·3	18·0	19·5	16·7	115	113

VI.—West Midland.												
Gloucestershire	31·5	29·6	46	43	1038	1034	18·7	18·4	19·8	17·1	129	127
Herefordshire	28 0	27·3	74	80	1028	1071	18·0	18·8	19·3	18·2	111	129
Shropshire	29·8	28·8	82	82	1047	1045	17·9	18·0	18·6	17·4	119	138
Staffordshire	39·2	36·1	48	49	1032	1017	20·8	19·4	20·0	18 2	153	158
Worcestershire	33·0	30·8	50	49	1027	1058	18·0	17·1	18·0	16·3	132	137
Warwickshire	35·9	32·3	40	41	1035	1036	20·1	19·1	20·3	17·9	149	156
VII.—North Midland.												
Leicestershire	36·4	34·3	48	48	1037	1044	19·9	19·2	20·7	17·8	165	173
Rutlandshire	30·6	27·5	50	54	1067	957	17·6	16·3	14·6	18·1	115	117
Lincolnshire	32·1	29·9	58	59	1045	1031	17·7	17·5	18·0	16·9	131	143
Nottinghamshire	37·4	35·9	60	57	1039	1036	20·4	19·5	20·5	18·5	157	166
Derbyshire	36·3	33·2	49	47	1043	1018	19·0	17·8	18·4	17·3	134	140
VIII.—North Western.												
Cheshire	33·8	31·9	51	52	1044	1036	19·9	18·7	19·6	17·9	139	146
Lancashire	36·9	33·7	45	46	1031	1040	23·3	21·9	23·1	20·7	163	174
IX.—Yorkshire.												
West Riding	35·6	31·4	51	52	1037	1026	21·1	19·1	20·1	18·1	155	155
East Riding (with York)	34·7	31·9	57	59	1017	1020	20·3	18·7	19·7	17·8	151	156
North Riding	35·7	31·9	59	59	1043	1041	18·6	17·0	17·3	16·5	133	135
X.—Northern.												
Durham	40·7	36·2	40	42	1044	1028	21·1	18·3	18·5	18·1	152	151
Northumberland	36·5	35·8	55	49	1039	1016	20·8	19·8	20·3	10·3	140	142
Cumberland	34·0	32·4	77	79	1043	1069	19·3	17·2	17·6	16·8	126	119
Westmoreland	30·4	28·8	74	69	1011	1129	16·7	14·7	15·7	13·7	104	88
XI.—Welsh.												
Monmouthshire	36·5	37·4	42	41	1042	1073	20·8	23·1	24·3	21·8	132	166
South Wales	35·2	34·9	46	42	1047	1056	19·9	21·0	22·2	19·9	131	158
North Wales	30·1	26·7	67	75	1012	1050	19·7	17·7	18·1	17·4	122	118

The influence of **Nationality** is shown in the following table:—

Birth-Rates per 1,000 Living in Different Countries.

Countries.	Mean Annual Birth-Rate in the 20 years 1861–80.	1881.	1882.	1883.	1884.	1885.	1886.	1887.
England and Wales	35·3	33·9	33·7	33·3	33·3	32·5	32·4	31·4
Scotland	34·9	33·7	33·3	32·5	33·4	32·3	32·4	31·2
Ireland	26·2 (17 yrs.)	24·5	24·1	23·6	24·0	23·5	23·3	23·2
Denmark	31·2	32·3	32·4	31·8	33·4	32·6	32·6	32·0
Norway	30·8 (10 yrs.)	30·0	30·9	30·9	31·0	31·3	30·9	—
Sweden	30·9	29·1	29·4	28·9	30·0	29·6	29·8	—
Austria	39·7	38·7	38·9	38·2	38·4	37·4	37·7	38·2
Hungary	42·8 (15 yrs.)	43·7	44·6	45·3	46 0	—	45·5	—
Switzerland . . .	30·6 (11 yrs.)	29·8	28·8	28·4	28·1	27·5	27·5	—
German Empire .	39·6 (9 yrs.)	37·0	37·2	36·6	37·2	37·0	37·1	36·9
Netherlands . . .	35·8	35·0	35·3	34·3	34·9	34·4	34 6	33·7
Italy	37·1 (18 yrs.)	38·0	37·1	37·1	38·7	38·1	36 1	35·3
France.	25·9	24·9	24·8	24·8	24·8	24·3	23 9	23·5

It will be seen that there is a general tendency to decrease of the birth-rate in the years for which registration is reliable. The decrease is much more marked in some countries than in others. In England and throughout Great Britain the decrease has been steady and uninterrupted. It may be ascribed to a smaller number of marriages (page 46), which doubtless has had some influence, or to diminished fecundity of each marriage, or to postponement of marriage to a later period of life, or to other causes; the relative importance of these different agencies being in fact somewhat doubtful.

The United States furnishes a good example of the difficulty encountered in estimating the true relative fecundity of the "native born" and immigrant population. The former comprises not only true Americans, but also the offspring of foreigners born in the States, and contains an excess of children; while the "foreign" population contains an excess of adults of reproductive ages. It is evident that the comparison of births per 1,000 of each population would not be fair. Such an erroneous method has led to the conclusion that foreigners are three or four times as prolific as the native-born population; whereas the difference which actually exists is much less marked. Thus the census of the State of Massachusetts for 1875 (quoted by Buck) showed that over 57 per cent. of the native-born women, twenty years of age and upwards, were mothers, and nearly 66 per cent. of foreigners of the same age.

Still-births are not registered in England; but under the new Registration Act no still-born child can be buried without a certificate from a registered practitioner in attendance, or from one who had examined the body, or a declaration from a midwife to the effect that the child was still-born. The proportion of still-births to total births in this country is supposed to be about 4 per cent., but this is uncertain. In France the children dying either before or after birth, if they die before registration, are recorded as still-born. This fact should be remembered in estimating the true death-rate and birth-rate of France. Thus the corrected death-rate of France in 1875 becomes 23·4 instead of 23·1 per 1,000 of population (Reg.-General's 38th Annual Report). The proper plan would be to register all still-births in a separate category, distinct from both births and deaths. The males outnumber females in still-births, probably owing to greater difficulty in childbirth. Thus in the ten years 1865–1875, they were in France, 144; Italy, 140; Belgium, 135; Sweden, 133; and in Prussia, 129 to every 100 female still-births.

Proportion of Males and Females at Birth.—The following table shows the proportion in successive groups of years in England and Wales:—

Years.	Males born to every 1,000 Females born.
In the ten years 1838–47	1050
,, ,, 1848–57	1046
,, ,, 1858–67	1044
,, ,, 1868–77	1039
,, six years 1878–83	1038
,, year 1884 . . .	1041
,, ,, 1885 . . .	1040
,, ,, 1886 . . .	1038
,, ,, 1887 . . .	1039

The proportion borne by male and female births during the ten years 1870–79, in different European countries, is shown in the following table:—

Country.	Males born to every 1,000 Females born.
Italy	1071
Austria	1068
France	1064
Switzerland	1063
German Empire . . .	1062
Holland	1061
Belgium	1059
Scotland	1057
Ireland	1056
England and Wales . .	1039

It will be seen that the proportion of boys to girls at birth is smaller in England than in any European country; while the preceding table (page 61) shows that for some unexplained reason the excess in the proportional number of boys is steadily decreasing. The proportion of boys to girls at birth in the various counties of England is shown in the table at page 58.

According to the "Upper Class" Table, there are at birth 1,053 boys to every 1,000 girls, and by the English Life Table of Dr. Farr, 1,048 to 1,000. The preponderance of males steadily diminishes with age, the diminution being most rapid in the first year of life. At the age of thirty-four, the two sexes are equal in number; after that, the diminution in the proportion of males goes on, until at the age of seventy, by the Upper Class Table they are 813, and by the English Life Table 925 to 1,000 females. The proportion of males is greater in large than in small families; it is greater also among the earlier born than the later born children in a family.

Illegitimacy has such important bearings on social problems, as well as on the chances of life of infants, that it deserves careful consideration.

It may be stated, (1) like the total death-rate, as a proportion to every 1,000 of the population.

(2) The most accurate method is to state it as a proportion to the number of unmarried women living at child-bearing ages. The number of both married and unmarried women of child-bearing years can be estimated from the census returns in the case of counties, and so their true rate of illegitimacy can be estimated.

(3) We may state it as a proportion to the total births, as in the table on page 58. This last method is somewhat fallacious, as the number of legitimate births varies with the marriage-rate, and this with the activity of trade; so that if the marriage-rate were low, and the number of illegitimate births remained stationary, the proportion of illegitimate to total births would appear larger than usual. Thus, in the year 1881, there were 4·9 illegitimate births to every hundred children born, a higher proportion than for the six preceding years, which was explained by the Registrar-General to be due, not to increase in the number of illegitimate births, but to diminution in the number of legitimate births, owing to a lower marriage-rate. That this was the true explanation is shown by the fact that the illegitimate birth-rate in 1881 (1·7 per 1,000 of the population) remained the same as in the six preceding years. It is therefore satisfactory that, notwithstanding the continued low marriage-rate, the illegitimate birth-rate was not affected thereby.

Illegitimate Birth-Rates.

Years.	Illegitimate Births to 1,000 Living.	Illegitimate Births in 1,000 Births.
1841–50	2·21	67
1851–60	2·23	65
1861–70	2·15	61
1871–80	1·76	50
1881	1·7	49
1882	1·6	49
1883	1·6	48
1884	1·6	47
1885	1·6	48
1886	1·5	47
1887	1·5	48

The same remarks apply even more for 1886–7, when the illegitimate birth-rate was the lowest on record.

Illegitimate births are more prone than legitimate births to escape registration, especially in populous districts. This deficiency of registration is probably on the decrease; but, spite of this, there is an uninterrupted and satisfactory decrease of total registered illegitimacy.

In *different counties* the proportion of illegitimate births varies greatly. In the table on pages 58, 59, they were 47 per 1,000 births, varying from 82 in Shropshire to 41 in Surrey, 34 in Essex, and 32 in Middlesex. The differences between various counties as regards the prevalence of illegitimacy remain very constant from year to year. The Registrar-General has pointed out that England and Wales can be not very roughly divided into three zones; a south zone with an illegitimate rate below the general average; a midland zone with illegitimacy somewhat above the average; and a northern zone with an excessively high rate of illegitimacy (see table, pages 58, 59). Shropshire always experiences an unenviable reputation in this respect. Thus, in 1885, while, roughly, 1 in 21 infants born in the whole country were born out of wedlock, in Shropshire the proportion was 1 in 11. It must not be assumed that the exact relative morality of different counties is undoubtedly stated by the figures in the table on pages 58, 59, on account of the fallacies to which we have previously alluded.

A considerable proportion of the illegitimate births occur *in workhouses*. Thus, in 1882, out of every 1,000 illegitimate births in England and Wales, 163 occurred in workhouses, while only 2·1 out of every 1,000 legitimate births occurred in these institutions. It is curious to note, that the proportion of illegitimate births in workhouses is greatest in those counties in which the illegitimate birth-rate is lowest, and conversely the proportion is lowest where there is a high rate of illegitimacy, possibly owing to more extensive and systematic domestic concubinage in the latter case.

Influence of Early Marriage on Illegitimacy.—The increasing number of early marriages during the ten years 1865–74 does not appear to have accounted for the decreasing rate of illegitimacy in England during the same period. This is shown by the following comparison made by Dr. Farr between the proportion born out of wedlock and the marriages under age in the four counties of Cumberland, Norfolk, Salop, and Westmoreland (in which illegitimacy was very high), with the same data for extra-metropolitan Middlesex and Surrey, London and Monmouth (in which illegitimacy was very low).

	Proportion per 100 Births born out of Wedlock.	Proportion per 100 Marriages under Age.	
		Men.	Women.
Cumberland, Norfolk, Salop, and Westmoreland.	9·6	5·7	17·5
Extra-metropolitan Middlesex and Surrey, London, and Monmouth.	8·0	5·0	18·2

This conclusion is confirmed by the fact that during the present decennium the proportion of marriages under age and the illegitimate birth-rate have both decreased.

Influence of Education on Illegitimacy.—There are few data bearing on this point; but the following table, abstracted from

Counties.	Births out of Wedlock to 100 Unmarried Women aged 15-55.	Percentage of Married Women who signed by Marks, 1851.
London	0·82	23
Devonshire . . .	1·12	36
Middlesex	1·17	30
Surrey	1·35	29
Cornwall	1·36	52
Sussex	1·54	29
Kent	1·62	34
England and Wales	1·72	45
Wiltshire	1·89	47
Lancashire . . .	1·90	63
Northumberland .	1·95	38
Cambridgeshire . .	2·01	46
Durham	2·02	48
West Riding . . .	2·09	59
Shropshire . . .	2·17	47
Staffordshire . . .	2·40	60
Norfolk	2·83	44

the Registrar-General's 14th Annual Report, shows the births out of wedlock in different parts of the country to 100 unmarried women aged 15–55, and in a parallel column the percentage of married women who signed the marriage register by marks in 1851.

The column giving the state of elementary education among married women throws indirect light on the state of education of the unmarried women; but it is evident that there is no uniform relationship between the state of education and amount of illegitimacy.

The Malthusian Hypothesis.—The "Essay on Population," by Malthus, the first edition of which appeared in 1798, has excited great criticism, both favourable and unfavourable; and as the opinions of Malthus have been espoused by eminent scientists, it becomes necessary to consider them carefully. For a fuller consideration of the subject, the reader should refer to Dr. Farr's Supplement to the 35th Annual Report of the Registrar-General, from which most of the facts hereafter stated have been obtained. The essay of Malthus was chiefly written to combat the views of Condorcet and Godwin, who held that the human race is advancing towards an ideal state of perfection. Malthus's conclusion was the exact opposite of this, the "principle of population," according to his contention, rendering vice and misery inevitable in all ages. He laid down the following principles, that (1) "population cannot increase without the means of subsistence," that (2) "population does invariably increase where there are the means of subsistence," and that (3) "the superior power of population cannot be checked without producing misery or vice." In a later edition he states that "the checks which repress the superior power of population, and keep its effects on a level with the means of subsistence, are all resolvable into moral restraint, vice, and misery." He further enunciated the doctrine, that "the population is increasing in a geometrical progression, the means of subsistence in an arithmetical progression; and unless wars, destructive epidemics, marshes, dense towns, close workshops, and other deadly agents, carry off the excess of the numbers born—unless the outlets of life and blood be left open—the whole people must be exposed to a slow process of starvation."

In this theory Malthus left out of account the fact that at child-bearing ages a large proportion of the population in every civilized country is unmarried and virtuous; only a partial recognition of this fact being given in the later editions of his work under the phrase "moral restraint." He insisted that the increase of mankind is the chief source of misery, and that the repression of population, or extensive celibacy, is a necessary condition of human happiness in the aggregate. He argued also that any decrease in the mortality from a given disease, as small-pox, must be accompanied by an increase in the mortality of some other diseases; and that great and ravaging epidemics are necessary, in the absence of war, to destroy what is redundant. It was but a corollary from this doctrine that Malthus should propose the plan that, after a given date, the poor laws should be abolished, and no child born from any marriage taking place after that date "should ever be entitled to parish assistance."

We may take each of Malthus's statements in turn, that (1) population increases in geometrical progression, while (2) the means of subsistence only increase in arithmetical progression.

Increase of Population in Geometrical Progression.—As shown on page 5, a population increases in geometrical progression when the births exceed the deaths, and the birth and death-rates remain constant. Thus, if the birth-rate were to remain 30·0 per 1,000, and its death-rate 19·0 per 1,000, the population would double itself in 63·4 years. But the numbers never actually increase, as the numbers in the geometrical series, 1, 2, 4, 8, 16, 32, indefinitely. As Farr points out, the principle of "an increase of the population in geometrical progression" has nothing in it irresistible or inexorable; it consists simply in an excess of births over the deaths, and becomes a "decrease of population in geometrical progression" if the births become fewer in number than the deaths; and the births may be reduced rapidly by retarding the period and number of marriages; so that the mathematical terror propounded by Malthus is purely theoretical.

The fact that one-fifth of the people of this country who attain the age of marriage never marry, and that women, although capable of bearing children at 16, do not marry until they attain a mean age of 24·7 (page 47), proves that "moral restraint" is in practical operation to an extent which is hardly realized.

Darwin applies the doctrine of Malthus to the whole vegetable and animal kingdom, and makes "the struggle for existence amongst all organic beings which inevitably follows from the high geometrical ratio of their increase" the basis of a vast generalization. He concludes that "all we can do is to keep steadily in mind that each organic being is striving to increase in a geometrical ratio; that each at some period of its life, during some season of the year, during each generation or at intervals, has to struggle for life and to suffer great destruction. When we reflect on this struggle, we may console ourselves with the full belief that the war of nature is not incessant, that no fear is felt, that death is generally prompt, and that the vigorous, the healthy, and the happy survive and multiply." This struggle doubtless reigns over the whole animal kingdom; but the presence of reason in man gives him certain prerogatives, by enabling him to control his fertility and ward off the blows of disease.

Increase of Subsistence in Arithmetical Progression.—The assumption that the increase of subsistence is in arithmetical progression will not bear examination. Subsistence—understanding by this term all that supplies men's wants—may for a certain number of years increase in geometrical progression. The productions of any country come under two natural divisions: (1) the natural produce of the earth, and (2) the portion which is created by human industry. The first of these corresponds to the food of animals, and is the only food available for savages. The second increases as the number of civilized men increases, and may be expected to continue to increase until the resources of science are exhausted. Malthus, however, throughout his work, loses sight of this necessary division, and confounds the natural and untilled yield of the earth with *the produce of human industry.* He also limits his view of produce to the single country occupied by the population under consideration, whereas, in virtue of the extension of trade, the resources of a country such as ours are drawn from every quarter of the globe. We have no exact valuation of the produce of this country at stated intervals. But money capital may be taken as representative of other working materials; and at compound interest its increase is much more rapid that that of any European population. Thus, at 3 per cent. per annum, compound interest, capital doubles itself in 24 years. A birth-rate of 3 per 100, which is near the actual present rate in England, would imply, in the absence of deaths, that the population would be doubled in the same period. But as the death-rate in 1886 was 1·9 per 100 of population, the real increase per 100, on the assumption that the birth-rate was 3 per 100, was 1·1, or ·011 per unit.

$$\text{Now } R^n = 2$$
$$(1{\cdot}011)^n = 2$$
$$n = \frac{\log 2}{\log 1{\cdot}011} = \frac{{\cdot}3010300}{{\cdot}0047512} = 63{\cdot}4 \text{ years.}$$

Therefore the population doubles itself in about 63 years, a much longer period than capital takes to double itself. The assertion that the disappearance of cholera or other epidemics must be followed by famine, or an increase of other diseases, falls to the ground. It may apply to the lower animals, like rabbits, who are dependent on the natural produce of the earth; but it is inapplicable to civilized man, who has the power of creating subsistence.

It has been already pointed out, that each member of the population, when the balance between expense of subsistence and wages earned through life is worked out, represents enormous wealth. It should be added, that if the Malthusian doctrine, which assumes that the restraint of population is the cornerstone of policy, were acted upon, it would lead to the annihilation of what is best in mankind, and we might never have had, for instance, a Robert Stephenson or a James Watt.

To the sanitarian, the Malthusian doctrine, which assumes the fewer the happier, is of the most serious import; for, if sanctioned, it must inevitably lead to relaxation of the efforts now being made to improve the condition of the public health. Only the most depraved would carry the doctrine so far as to propose the actual destruction of life; but its advocates are logically bound to welcome a high infantile mortality, and to regard the large destruction of juvenile life by such diseases as whooping cough and measles with complacency, while efforts to remove insanitary conditions and obviate unhealthy employments must be regarded as an attempt to evade the action of an inevitable and, from their standpoint, a beneficial law. We shall find later that *the births almost invariably increase when the mortality increases ;* where the mortality is greatest the population is multiplying most rapidly; and that thus an increase of mortality is by no means the specific for the cure of over-population which Malthus considered it to be (page 84).

Influence of Birth-rate on Age-Constitution of Population.—The age-distribution of a population, *i.e.*, the relative number of persons living at different groups of ages, depends principally upon the rate of increase of the population (page 73). This increase may be due to excess of births over deaths (natural increase) or to immigration. Immigration is generally of comparatively young adults, and thus has an important bearing on the death-rate, which it tends to lower. A population such as that of England, with a birth-rate persistently higher than the death-rate, contains an undue proportion of children, of youths, and of persons of middle life, and, as in the case of immigration, there results a lowering of the death-rate. The undue proportion of persons of a lower age may be explained as follows: In a stationary population undisturbed by migration, the number of births equals the number of deaths, and if the rate of mortality at different ages does not vary from time to time and the births and deaths are uniformly distributed throughout each year, the

DIAGRAM OF THE POPULATION OF
ENGLAND & WALES AT DIFFERENT AGES AS ENUMERATED IN THE YEAR, 1871.

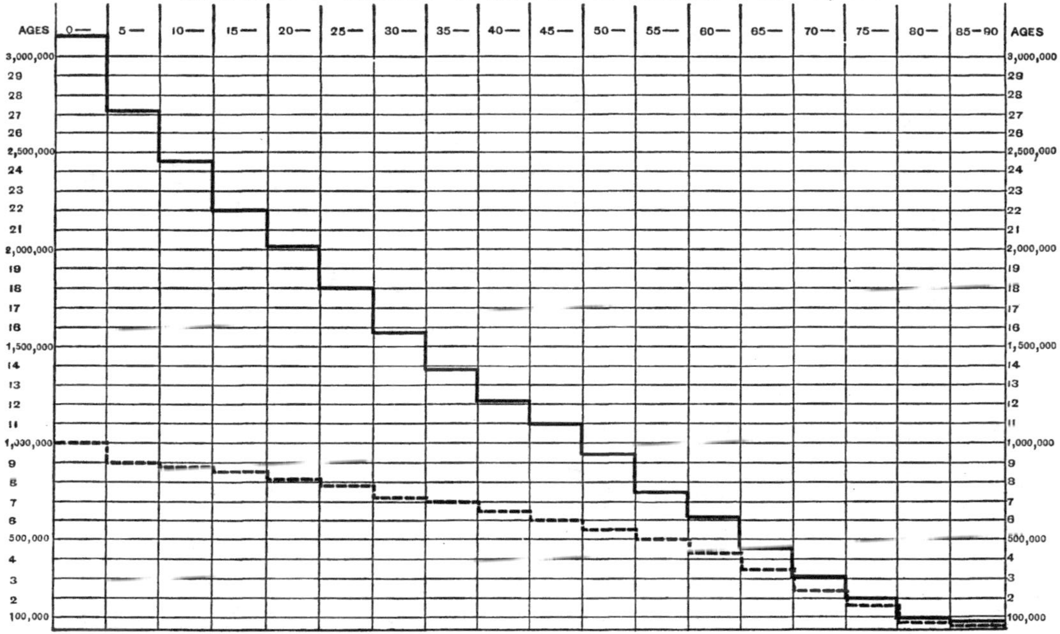

The Diagram ***represents*** *by its area enclosed by the continuous dark line, the relative numbers of the Population* ***in*** 18 *groups of ages, as enumerated at the Census of* 1871. *The area enclosed by the dotted lower line represents what the population would have been had the births remained uniformly* 253,320 *a year, as in* 1771, *instead of increasing as they did to* 797,428 *in* 1871. *Thus in the population as enumerated in* 1871, 3,100,000 *children were living who were under the age of* 5 *years, while in the population with the stationary number of births the number of children of that age would be one million only.*

age-constitution of the population remains uniform. The births and deaths in the stationary population being equal in number, the birth- and death-rates are also identical. If now the birth-rate suddenly increases, the number living in the first year of life will increase; and if this higher birth-rate persists, in the second year of its occurrence the number living under two years of age will be increased, in the third year the number living under three years, and so on. If the high birth-rate continues for, say, 40 years, the number living at all ages under 40 will be increased, and so on. But for about twenty of these forty years a further influence will have been brought to bear. Those aged 20–40 who were born under the conditions of the hypothesis have children of their own; so that, assuming the birth-rate to remain stationary, the *absolute number of births* per annum is increasing rapidly every year. The consequence of this uninterrupted increase in the annual number of births is, that the proportion of those living at the earlier ages as compared with the entire population becomes greater, and a distribution of the population is arrived at which we shall find is favourable to a low death-rate (page 84).

The disturbing effect on the age of a population of a yearly increasing number of births is shown in the accompanying diagram from the supplement to the Registrar-General's 35th Annual Report (page 73).

We have assumed in the preceding remarks, that the change was from a stationary population to one with a birth-rate higher than its death-rate, but in which the birth-rate remained constant after it had once increased. If, however, the birth-rate were continuously to increase, the effect in disturbing the normal or Life-Table distribution of a population would be still greater, and for many years this was the state of things in England. In the last few years, however, the birth-rate has decreased, and, as shown by the following figures, there is but a very slight increase in the absolute number of births. Such a condition of the factors producing population will obviously have a much less disturbing influence on its age-distribution than if the number of births were continuously to increase.

If the total annual births were to remain stationary in number, the disturbance in the age-distribution of the population would, as the wave of population advances, gradually disappear.

Now, a high mortality depresses the average age of those living, owing to the fact that the mortality steadily increases

Year.	Number of Births.	Birth-Rate.
1880	881,643	34·2
1881	883,642	33·9
1882	889,014	33·7
1883	890.722	33·3
1884	906,750	33·3
1885	894,270	32·5
1886	903,866	32·4
1887	886,331	31·4

with advance of years. It follows that, as the death-rate is low in England, its people should on an average be older than elsewhere. But the increased number of births during the last century has so increased the proportion of children and young persons that it may be doubted whether the people of any other country are so young as those of England and Scotland. The exact relationship between birth-rate and death-rate will be discussed at page 84.

Natural Increase of Population.—The *natural increment* of a population in any year equals the births *minus* the deaths. It may be greater, owing either to a diminished number of deaths or an increased number of births. The *actual increment* is governed also by the balance between immigration and emigration, and we have not the necessary data for determining it accurately during each year. During the ten years 1871–80 the natural increment amounted to 3,425,982, and the actual increment, as determined by the census, amounted to 3,256,020. Thus in the ten years there was a loss by the excess of emigration over immigration of 169,962 persons, which loss consisted of 138,324 males and 31,638 females. The

Registrar-General has therefore adopted the method (which, in the absence of more frequent census enumerations, seems the least open to objection) of assuming that the rate of growth which existed in the last intercensal period has been maintained in the years which have since elapsed.

A stationary rate of natural increase might occur under the following different conditions: (1) if the birth-rate and death-rate both increased to a corresponding extent; (2) if the birth-rate and death-rate both decreased to a corresponding extent. It is the difference between the birth- and death-rates which governs the result. Thus in 1883 the natural increase of the population of England and Wales was lower than in the previous year, a result which was due, not to increased mortality (the death-rate falling slightly in 1883), but to a decline in the birth-rate from 33·7 in 1882 to 33·3 in 1883.

Similarly in 1881 there was a high natural increase, owing not to a high birth-rate (which was the lowest since 1851), but to a great diminution in the deaths, which in this year were only 1 in 53 of the population, the lowest record in any previous year being 1 in 49. In 1882, on the other hand, there was a falling-off in the natural increase, not due to a diminution in births, but to an increase in the number of deaths.

Year.	Natural Increase.	Natural Increase per 1,000 of Population.	Births per 1,000 of Population.	Deaths per 1,000 of Population.
1880	353,019	13·7	34·2	20·5
1881	391,707	15·2	33·9	18·9
1882	372,360	14·3	33·7	19·6
1883	367,725	13·8	33·3	19·5
1884	375,922	13·9	33·3	19·5
1885	371,520	13·6	32·5	19·0
1886	366,590	13·2	32·4	19·3
1887	355,573	12·6	31·4	18·8

From the rate of natural increase we can obtain directly the time required for the population to double itself. Thus, in

1886 the rate of natural increase per 1,000 was 13·2 = ·0132 per unit.

Now $M = P \cdot R^n$, where, as in compound interest,

M = amount when increased = principal + interest.

P = principal = original population.

$R = 1 +$ rate of increase per unit.

r = rate of increase per unit.

$R = 1 + r$.

n = number of years.

Required, the time required to double the population.

Call $M = 2$, and $P = 1$.

Then $2 = 1 \times R^n = R^n = (1 + r)^n$.

$= (1 + \cdot 0132)^n = (1 \cdot 0132)^n$.

$\therefore$ Log. $2 = n$ log. $1 \cdot 0132$.

$$\therefore\ n = \frac{\log.\ 2}{\log.\ 1\cdot 0132} = \frac{301030}{\cdot 005694} = \mathbf{52 \cdot 8}\ \text{years.}$$

CHAPTER VI.

DEATHS.

Estimation of Death-rate.—Death-rates for Short Periods.—General and Special Death-rates.—Effect of Migration on Death-rate.—Correction for Visitors.—Effect of Public Institutions.—Influence of Birth-rate on Death-rate.—Opposite Views of Letheby and Farr.—Influence of Age and Sex-distribution on Death-rate.—Proportion of Males and Females in Population.—Method of Correction for Age and Sex-distribution.—Standard, Recorded, and Corrected Death-rates.—Factors for Correction.—Trustworthiness of General Death-rates.

MORTALITY statistics surpass all others in importance, whether they are considered from a social, or actuarial, or sanitary standpoint. We must therefore consider them in detail.

Estimation of Death-Rate.—The death-rate may be reckoned (1) in proportion to every thousand of the mean population; or (2) the proportion of deaths, taken as unity, to the whole population may be stated. Thus, in 1886 the death-rate per 1,000 was 19·3, which is equivalent to 1 in 51.

The two are easily convertible by division.

$$\frac{1{,}000}{51} = 19{\cdot}3. \frac{1{,}000}{19{\cdot}3} = 51.$$

Death-Rates for Short Periods.—It is evident that the shorter the period to which a death-rate refers the greater the liability to error, owing to accidental causes of variation. But the death-rate for a short period expresses a fact, the errors only arising when we draw wide inferences from facts relating to short periods. Large fluctuations from accidental causes occur especially in connection with small populations. A temporary high death-rate may, for instance, only mean that, owing to the prevalence of inclement weather, a considerable number of unstable and fragile lives have had their deaths slightly hastened.

The *death-rates for each week* published by the Registrar-General are *annual* death-rates per 1,000 of the mean population of the year; *i.e.*, they represent the number who would die per 1,000 of the population, supposing the same proportion of deaths to population held good throughout the year. They are, therefore, not actual rates at all, and the public should be warned against the indiscriminate use of them for comparison. They may be of service in contrasting with the death-rate of the same place at the corresponding period of a preceding year, and as showing the influence of seasonal variations; but should be received with caution when used to compare one town with another.

The death-rate for a week might be obtained, if there were exactly 52 weeks in a year, by multiplying the deaths by 52, or dividing the population by 52, and then proceeding as for an annual death-rate. But the correct number of days in a natural year is 365·24226, and the correct number of weeks therefore 52·17747. The Registrar-General therefore divides, for the purposes of his weekly returns, the estimated population of each town by 52·17747, thus obtaining what may be called the weekly population of the town. Thus, if the population of a town is 143,956, its weekly population is

$$\frac{143,956}{52{\cdot}17747}=2,758,$$

which is assumed to remain constant for the year for which the calculation is required. Now, if there are 35 deaths in one week; then the annual death-rate for the week in question

$$=\frac{35\times 1,000}{2758}=12{\cdot}69$$

It would be more logical to multiply the deaths of each week by 52·17747 than to deal with the population; but as this would require to be done each week, the former method is evidently less laborious, and produces the same results.

The Registrar-General makes his death-rates *for each*

quarter refer to the thirteen weeks most nearly corresponding with the natural quarter; and the quarterly population is obtained by multiplying by thirteen the population of one week.

The death-rate, expressing the proportion borne by deaths from all causes to each thousand of the population, is known as the **general** or **crude death-rate.** The fallacies detracting from its value as a test of relative vitality will be subsequently considered. It should be regarded as the first test, to be followed up by further research. It is doubtful, however, whether, in the case of large populations, any more trustworthy test is available; and its value may be regarded as remaining unimpaired, spite of numerous attacks upon it.

Special death-rates are also employed; and these may be divided into two kinds: (1) those which differentiate the persons affected as to age and sex, race, social condition, occupation, density of population, locality, season, etc.; and (2) those which differentiate the causes of mortality, as zymotic diseases, phthisis, violence, suicide, etc.

We can only discuss in this chapter the influence on the death-rate of movements of the population, of large institutions, of the birth-rate, and of the age and sex distribution of the population.

Effect of Movements of Population.—The effect produced by immigration and emigration will vary in proportion to the average age and sex of the migrants. The mortality of most large and growing towns would stand higher than it does but for the large number of young and healthy immigrants from the country. Similarly, watering-places and residential towns appear somewhat healthier than they are, because of the large proportion of young domestic servants.

The low death-rate of New Zealand—12·4 per 1,000 for the years 1866–75—was doubtless due partly to its equable climate and the prosperous condition of its population; but much more to the constant stream of mostly young immigrants, and to its high birth-rate.

The bulk of the immigrants to towns are probably in good

health; but a certain number go from the country into the town hospitals. On the other hand, many townspeople suffering from phthisis or other chronic disease migrate into the country, and aged persons very commonly do the same.

Dr. Ransome has proposed not to calculate the deaths over fifteen years of age, as being affected by migration, but to compare the death-rate of various towns for ages under fifteen. This might be suitable for Manchester, but not for other towns. Thus seaside towns like Margate and Brighton, which have a large number of boarding-schools, would be unfairly represented.

The only way to avoid the fallacies arising from this cause would be to have records kept of the movements of population, and the births and deaths of each place subjected to analysis before comparison is made. In order that the death-rates of two populations should be comparable on equal terms, so far as migration is concerned, it would be necessary that (*a*) the number of immigrants and the average duration of their residence should balance the number of emigrants and the average duration of their absence; and that (*b*) the proportion of sexes living at each age, their state of health and liability to disease, should be the same among both.

Such conditions are not attainable even in European States, where a record of migrants is kept, and much less so in this country; and it is satisfactory to remember, therefore, that in most instances the sources of mistake tend to counteract each other; and the most important fallacy, that arising from varying age-distribution of the population, can be avoided by giving the death-rate separately for different groups of ages.

There is another way in which migration may affect mortality statistics. In the case of districts inhabited by *artisans and labourers*, there is always an extraneous population pressing in to fill the vacuum caused by removal or death, so that, as pointed out in regard to Liverpool by Dr. French in 1865, the same house may in one year represent the accidents, deaths, and diseases of twenty-four persons, instead of the six persons which the census gives for each house. This is analogous to the error in *hospital statistics*, when the number of deaths per bed (the *bed death-rate*) is given as an estimate of the relative mortality and sanitary condition of different hospitals and infirmaries. Of course the chances of death are increased in proportion to the number of times a house or a bed is occupied during the year. In a less degree, the same remarks may apply to a town subject to frequent *ingress of visitors*, the chances of death increasing with the frequency that the population of the town undergoes change.

The following remarks from a local report of my own give a good example of the difficulties in estimating the true death-rate in a town where the visitors at certain times of the year increase the population of 143,956 by as much as 50,000 persons:—

"The fact that the population of Brighton is, during the greater part of the year, swollen by the ingress of thousands of visitors, of whose number we have no trustworthy estimate, and who yet furnish a quota to its mortality, makes a true calculation of the death-rate per thousand of the population a difficult matter. My predecessor, Dr. Taaffe, estimated that an addition of 10,000 to the resident population would represent the average number of visitors in Brighton. It should be remembered, however, that the census enumerations in April, 1871 and 1881 (which form the basis of calculation of the population for the current year), necessarily included all the visitors present at those dates, and that Brighton benefits by the very slightly lowered death-rate which these additions to its population involve. It must be added, however, that there is probably no time of year in which the number of visitors in Brighton is at so low an ebb as in April (when the national census is taken).

"So far as population is concerned, the course theoretically least open to objection is *to exclude any estimated population of visitors and all deaths of visitors* in calculating the true death-rate of Brighton.

"I append a comparative table of death-rates for recent years; those in the first column being the *crude* death-rates as given by the Registrar-General, and those in the second column being the death-rates calculated on the number of deaths excluding deaths of visitors, and the population excluding all visitors except the small number included in the resident April population, which latter I can suggest no means of eliminating. The death-rates in the second column are consequently too small, though this deficiency cannot exceed 0·5 per 1,000 inhabitants."

Year.	Crude Death-Rate.	Death-Rate excluding visitors.
1882	21·6	20·4
1883	19·2	17·9
1884	18·0	16·7
1885	17·1	15·7
1886	17·1	16·1
1887	16·3	15·9

Effect of Public Institutions.—The consideration of the effect public institutions exert on local bills of mortality naturally follows on a consideration of the effect of migrations, as the inequality arising from such institutions is due to migrations into them from outlying districts. The rule in dealing with a public institution is to deduct the deaths of those inmates derived from outside the district concerning which the calculation is made, at the same time including the deaths of inhabitants of the said district which may have occurred in other institutions outside the district. Thus, Workhouses and Asylums are often situated outside the district from which they receive inmates; and in London and other great towns the large public hospitals receive patients from outlying districts. The deaths in all these cases must be relegated to their respective districts.

Thus, during the three months ending Sept. 30th, 1888, there were 71 deaths in the public institutions of Brighton (hospitals and workhouse). The total number of deaths in Brighton during the same period was 416—*i.e.*, 345 in private houses, and 71 in public institutions.

Of the deaths in private houses 7 were of visitors.
" " institutions 12 " "
Deaths excluding visitors $=416-19=397$.

Now the quarterly population of the municipal borough of Brighton $=29{,}996$.

Therefore the annual death-rate $=\dfrac{397\times 1000}{29{,}996}=\mathbf{13{\cdot}23}$.

A more difficult case is that of the Wandsworth sub-district of the Wandsworth District (London, S.W.). This sub-district has within its borders the County Lunatic Asylum, the Hospital for Incurables, St. Peter's Hospital, Wandsworth Prison, and the Royal Patriotic Asylum for Girls; and it sends its sick poor to the Wandsworth and Clapham Workhouse Infirmary, which is outside its borders, while some of its inhabitants die in the large metropolitan hospitals.

Total deaths in Wandsworth in 1885 were	628
Of these there occurred in its internal institutions . .	132

In addition there occurred in the Union Infirmary and other outlying Institutions 78 deaths.

The mean population of Wandsworth in 1885 was 31,497.

(1) The death-rate, uncorrected for internal institutions, and not including outlying institutions, is $\dfrac{628\times 1{,}000}{31{,}497}=19{\cdot}83$ per thousand.

(2) In order to ascertain the death-rate corrected for internal institutions without including the deaths in outlying institutions, we must ascertain the *population of its institutions* as well as their *deaths*. By the census of 1881 this was 1,482, which may be taken as nearly correct for 1885.

Corrected population $=31{,}497-1{,}482=30{,}015$.
Corrected deaths $=628-132=496$.

$$\text{Death-rate}=\frac{496\times 1{,}000}{30{,}015}=16{\cdot}52.$$

(3) The death-rate excluding the population and deaths of internal institutions, and including the deaths (but not the population, because this is unknown) of Wandsworth parishioners in outlying institutions.

Population = 30,015.

Deaths = 496 + 78 = 574.

$$\text{Death-rate} = \frac{574 \times 1{,}000}{30{,}015} = 19{\cdot}12.$$

The last death-rate more nearly than any other represents the true mortality of the Wandsworth sub-district. For it excludes the population and deaths in its numerous internal institutions (to which Wandsworth contributes only an inappreciable quota); and it allows for the deaths of Wandsworth parishioners in external institutions. The only fallacy is, that no allowance is made in the population for those inhabitants of Wandsworth who are in the outlying institutions without their illness proving fatal. This number must, however, be comparatively small, and cannot very materially affect the result.

Each Sanitary Authority in London is supplied quarterly from the Registrar-General's office with particulars of deaths of their inhabitants in outlying institutions, so that the necessary correction can be made. In provincial towns, however, there is reason to believe that such corrections are commonly avoided. A lunatic asylum or workhouse outside the borders of the town receives patients from it, but its mortality is steadily ignored. On the other hand, the mortality of many rural districts is lowered by the fact that many poorer people when ill become inmates of the neighbouring town hospital and there die. No just reason exists why these deaths should not be fairly stated, and we may hope that public opinion will in time demand this.

Influence of Birth-rate on Death-rate.—The influence of the birth-rate on the increase of the population and on the age-constitution of the population has been already considered. The age-constitution of the population has a most important bearing on the death-rate, which it may considerably modify; the birth-rate affecting the death-rate only in so far as it alters the age-constitution of the population.

Great fallacies are involved in the question of the relation between the birth-rate and death-rate. The two are assumed to be connected in two different ways. (1) A high birth-rate causes a high death-rate, and a low birth-rate causes a low death-rate. (2) The exact converse of this holds good, the death-rate controlling the birth-rate.

The interpretation of the true relationship between the birth-rate and death-rate depends on an appreciation of what has been said (page 70) concerning the influence of the birth-rate on the age-constitution of a population. It is evident that if, owing to a high birth-rate, there is a larger proportion of children in one community than in another, and the relative sanitary conditions of the two are equal, there will be more deaths of children in the former; and inasmuch as the rate of mortality of young children is higher than that of all others except the aged, the general death-rate will be raised. But if the high birth-rate be *continued*, there will not only be a large proportion of children, but of others between 10 and 40 years of age, at which ages a low rate of mortality holds; and this factor counterbalances the other, and makes a continued high birth-rate produce a low death-rate. Thus, speaking generally, the mortality of a population in which there is an excess of births over deaths is lower than that of a stationary population, in which the births and deaths are equal in number; the reason being on reflection obvious. In the latter case there is a larger proportion of old people than in the former. The rule therefore is, that *the lower the average age of a population* (mean age of living) *the lower ought to be its death-rate.*

The late Dr. Letheby may be regarded as the spokesman of those who take a view diametrically opposed to that just stated. He held that "the birth-rate is the controlling element of the death-rate"; that "an increase in the rate of mortality is often a sign of prosperity, for a high death-rate means a high birth-rate, and a high birth-rate is the invariable concomitant of prosperity." According to this view, a high birth-rate is a direct cause of a high death-rate, owing to the great mortality among infants We have, however, following the lines of Dr. Farr's argument, shown the fallacy of this theory, ignoring as it does the important fact that a continuously high birth-rate not only causes an excess of the infantile population, among whom the mortality is great, but also an excess of persons between 10 and 40 years of age, among whom the mortality is low.

Birth-Rates and Death-Rates in 1887.

Towns.	Birth-Rate	Death-Rate.
Brighton	25·8	16·9
Derby	30·0	17·1
Nottingham	33·3	18·7
50 Large Town Districts	32 2	19·0
Hull	32·8	19·2
Leicester	32·8	19·5
Portsmouth	36·8	19·5
London	31·7	19·6
Birmingham	31·8	19·7
Sunderland	34·6	19·7
Edinburgh	29·3	19·8
Bradford	27·7	19·9
Norwich	33·9	20·4
Bristol	29·7	20·4
28 Great Towns	32·2	20·8
Birkenhead	32·5	21·0
Halifax	28·4	21·0
Leeds	33·3	21·1
Bolton	32 5	21·3
Sheffield	32·9	21·6
Wolverhampton	33·2	21·7
Cardiff	41·1	21·9
Berlin	32·6	21·9
Amsterdam	36·6	22·1
Salford	31·9	22·2
Plymouth	31·5	22·7
Huddersfield	27·7	23·0
Glasgow	37·0	23·2
Paris	27·2	23·4
Liverpool	31·2	23·7
Oldham	31·3	23·8
Newcastle	39·1	25·3
Blackburn	35·8	25 5
Bombay	20·0	26·3
New York	23·0	26·4
Preston	38·5	27·9
Manchester	35·9	28·7
Dublin	28·0	30·6
Madras	41·2	40·3

That a high birth-rate and a high death-rate commonly coexist is certain, though the concurrence is by no means constant nor do the variations in the two follow on equal lines, as shown in the preceding table, in which the towns are arranged in order of their death-rates (page 85).

If a high birth-rate is necessarily followed by a high death-rate, the former must be regarded as an indication of a low sanitary condition. It is difficult to believe, however, that an increase of reproductive power argues a depression of vitality. The greater fertility in crowded districts is explained by the much higher proportion of people at child-bearing ages, owing to the inrush of young workers in search of the higher town wages. That there should be a high death-rate in such populations is in spite and not in consequence of the high birth-rate; and the high death-rate is due in reality to density of population and its concomitant social and sanitary evils. When a high death-rate follows a high birth-rate, it is due largely to *excessive infantile mortality*. Infants form a delicate index to the sanitary status of a population.

Low birth-rates and low death-rates also usually coexist. But the conclusion that one causes the other is altogether untenable. In France there is a low birth-rate and a high death-rate, owing largely to the fact that the continuous low birth-rate has caused the average age of the population to be considerably higher than in this country. On the other hand, in Staffordshire and Durham, in which the excess of births over deaths is very great, the death-rate is by no means the highest (see table, page 58).

To sum up: Dr. Farr has clearly shown that populations having a continuously high birth-rate, should (sanitary conditions being equal) have lower death-rates than populations having low birth-rates, because a continuously high birth-rate means an exceptionally large proportion of young adults in a population, and consequently an unduly small proportion of old people. Conversely, a low birth-rate means a small proportion of young adults and a large proportion of adults and old people, and is therefore unfavourable to a low death-rate.

The same conclusions are clearly demonstrated by Mr. N. A.

Humphreys, in his paper on "The Value of Death-Rates as a Test of Sanitary Condition." He takes as examples the birth and death-rates of three agricultural and three urban counties in 1871, and finds the *normal death-rate* in the two groups by allowing for varying age-distribution. The result is shown in the following table :—

	Three Agricultural Counties.	Three Urban Counties.
Birth-Rate	30·6	39·2
Death Rate	20·0	26·9
Normal or Life-Table Death-Rate	23·8	22·0

It might be assumed that the higher death-rate of the urban counties is explained by their higher birth-rate; but when correction is made for different age-constitution of the two populations, it is seen that, all sanitary conditions being equal, the age-constitution of the urban populations favours their death-rate to the extent of 1·8 per 1,000, instead of in any way explaining the high death-rate, as maintained by Dr. Letheby and others.

Influence of Age and Sex-Distribution on Death-Rate.—We shall consider at this point the modifications in the general death-rate which may result from varying age and sex-constitution of a population, reserving to the next chapter the consideration of death-rates at different ages.

Dr. Ogle has summed up the matter in the following words: "It is necessary to point out that two places might be on a perfect equality with each other as regards their climate, their sanitary arrangements, their closeness of aggregation, as also the habits and occupations of their inhabitants, and yet might have very different general death-rates, owing to differences in the age and sex-distribution of their respective populations. Such a supposed case is, of course, scarcely likely to present itself; for when the prevalent occupations are the same in two places, the age and sex-distribution is almost certain to be the same also. But in places where the prevalent occupations are not the same, there are often very great differences in the age and sex-distribution of the populations, and such as seriously affect the general death-rates."

The age and sex-distribution in any district determine mainly the prevalent occupations; and as the occupations remain fairly constant, the age and sex-distribution likewise vary but little. Thus no difficulty arises in comparing the death-rate of the same district or town at different periods. It is only when different districts or towns are compared that the necessity for correction (and ofttimes considerable correction) arises. The differences due to varying sex-distribution are usually very small, and it therefore generally suffices to correct for age-distribution.

In order to appreciate the influence on the death-rate of varying age and sex-distribution, we must examine the death-rates at different age-groups and in the two sexes. These are shown for four decennia in the following table from Dr. Ogle's Supplement to the 45th Annual Report of the Registrar-General:—

Annual Mortality per 1,000 *of Males and Females in successive Decennia.*

	Males.				Females.			
	1841-50.	1851-60.	1861-70.	1871-80.	1841-50.	1851-60	1861-70.	1871-80.
All Ages . .	23·11	23·05	23·61	22·61	21·58	21·32	21·28	20·00
Under 5 years	71·20	72·43	73·16	68·14	61·09	62·74	63·43	58·10
5–	9·16	8·51	8·15	6·67	8·89	8·42	7·76	6·20
10–	5·12	4·88	4·46	3·69	5·42	5·06	4·48	3·70
15–	7·05	6·69	6·16	5·23	7·88	7·38	6·62	5·43
20–	9·50	8·83	8·45	7·32	9·08	8·53	7·96	6·78
25–	9·94	9·57	9·90	9·30	10·55	9·92	9·68	8·58
35–	12·85	12·48	13·46	13·74	12·91	12·15	12·03	11·58
45–	18·22	17·96	19·16	20·05	16·04	15·20	15·55	15·59
55–	31·81	30·85	33·00	34·76	28·44	27·01	27·77	28·54
65–	67·51	65·33	66·69	69·57	60·97	58·66	58·80	60·82
75 & upwards	168·56	165·40	164·64	169·08	157·89	155·45	154·28	155·83

The table shows that between the ages of five and fifty-five the death-rate per 1,000 living at each group of ages is lower than the death-rate for all ages. It is evident, therefore, that an unusually large proportion of persons living at these ages would be a cause of low mortality. Under five and over fifty-five the death-rate is higher than the death-rate for all ages; and an excess of population at these ages would consequently raise the general death-rate.

The age-distribution of populations is therefore of great importance in determining the relative value of their death-rates. If they are identical in two localities, then any differences in their death-rates may be referred to influences peculiar to each place. As Farr puts it, "Independently of other causes of variation, the mortality of different populations will differ according as they consist of numbers in various proportions at the ages at which the mortality is high or low." The same reasoning applies for sex-distribution. At nearly all ages the death-rate of females is lower than that of males. Consequently an excess of females (as in residential neighbourhoods with a large number of domestic servants) must tend to lower the death-rate of a district, without implying a necessarily better sanitary condition.

Number of Males living to every 100 *Females living* (*exclusive of the portion of the Army, Navy, and Merchant Seamen abroad*).

Census Years.	Number of Males living in England and Wales to 100 Females.
Mean of 1821–31	96·35
,, 1831–41	95·87
,, 1841–51	95·80
,, 1851–61	95·51
,, 1861–71	94·96
,, 1871–81	94·84

The preceding table shows that, spite of the excess of male

births, females preponderate in the entire population. This excess of females in the English population would be still larger but for the large proportion of the population living at the earlier ages, when the number of males considerably exceeds that of females. The proportion of the two sexes would be somewhat altered if the number of Englishmen engaged abroad in the army, navy, and merchant service were taken into account. The differences of mortality due to variations in sex-distribution are usually so small that they may be in practice neglected.

The distribution of the population as to age and sex favours a low mortality—

(1) In newly settled communities.

(2) In towns, and especially when they are rapidly increasing; and

(3) In manufacturing as compared with agricultural neighbourhoods.

The high mortality which usually holds in such populations would be still higher but for their favourable age and sex-constitution.

Dr. Ransome gives an example which may serve to illustrate differences in the general rate of mortality, due simply to varying age-distribution of population. Suppose two towns, *A* and *B*, each with 1,000 inhabitants, and exactly alike in their sanitary conditions. *A* has 150 children under five; *B* has only 100 under five, which in each case die at the rate of 10 per cent. per annum, while persons over five die at the rate of 10 per mille. Reckoning up the total mortality per 1.000 at all ages, we find that

In *A*, out of 150 children, 15 die.
„ „ 850 over 5, 8·5 die; equal to 23·5 per 1,000 of the entire population.

In *B*, out of 100 children, 10 die.
„ „ 900 over 5, 9 die; equal to 19·0 per 1,000.

Thus there is a difference of 4·5 per 1,000 in the death-rate, due simply to differences in the composition of the two populations, and apart altogether from their state of health.

Dr. Ransome further points out that a death-rate of ten or even twelve per 1,000, which is not infrequently recorded in certain favoured districts, cannot be regarded as a true measure of longevity of its inhabitants. A death-rate of ten per 1,000 means either that every child born attains the age of one hundred before he dies, or else that the average age at death is one hundred, and that if some die in infancy, others must have lived much more than a hundred. Similarly, a death-rate of twelve per 1,000 means an average age at death of over eighty. "Under present conditions such figures are not attained by any community in the world, and can only be looked for in the millennium, when, as Isaiah says, the child shall die an hundred years old."

There are only two ways of avoiding the fallacies involved in unequal age and sex-constitution of populations submitted to comparison:

(1) The method to be immediately described; and

(2) A statement of the death-rate at various groups of ages, and in the two sexes, as given in the next chapter.

Method of Correction for Age and Sex-Distribution.—The Registrar-General described, in his Annual Summary for 1883, the method of correcting the death-rates in the twenty-eight great towns, giving in parallel columns the recorded and corrected death-rates for each town. This has been continued for subsequent years, and I append the table for 1887, the towns being arranged in the order of their corrected death-rates.

Towns in the order of their Corrected Death-rates.	Standard Death-rate.	Factor for Correction for Age and Sex-Distribution.	Recorded Death-rate.	Corrected Death-rate.	Comparative Mortality Figure.
Cols.	1.	2.	3.	4.	5.
England and Wales .	—	1·0000	18·78	18·78	1,000
England and Wales, less the 28 towns .	—	—	17·79	17·40	927
28 Towns	19·96	1·0657	20·83	22·20	1,182
Brighton	20·66	1·0296	16·88	17·38	925
Derby	20·45	1·0402	17·13	17·82	949
Norwich	22·24	0·9565	20·44	19·55	1,041
Nottingham . . .	20·07	1·0599	18·71	19·83	1,056
Hull	20·62	1·0316	19·25	19·86	1,058
Portsmouth . . .	20·65	1·0301	19·51	20·10	1,070
Leicester	20·31	1·0474	19·52	20·45	1,089
Sunderland . . .	20·43	1·0412	19·72	20·53	1,093
London	20·04	1·0615	19·57	20·77	1,106
Birmingham . . .	19·95	1·0663	19·72	21·03	1,120
Bristol	20·55	1·0351	20·39	21·11	1,124
Bradford	19·26	1·1045	19·93	22·01	1,172
Wolverhampton . .	20·63	1·0311	21·67	22·34	1,190
Birkenhead	19·89	1·0695	20·99	22·45	1,195
Leeds	19·90	1·0689	21·06	22·51	1,199
Plymouth	21·48	0·9903	22·74	22·52	1,199
Halifax	19·58	1·0864	20·95	22·76	1,212
Sheffield	19·78	1·0754	21·60	23·23	1,237
Bolton	19·41	1·0959	21·31	23·35	1,243
Cardiff	19·60	1·0853	21·92	23·79	1,267
Salford	19·54	1·0886	22·15	24·11	1,284
Huddersfield . . .	19·37	1·0982	22·99	25·25	1,345
Liverpool	19·39	1·0971	23·70	26·00	1,384
Oldham	19·17	1·1097	23·84	26·46	1,409
Newcastle	20·10	1·0583	25·26	26·73	1,423
Blackburn	19·52	1·0898	25·48	27·77	1,479
Preston	19·59	1·0859	27·92	30·32	1,614
Manchester	19·09	1·1143	28·67	31·95	1,701

In the preceding table the *standard death-rate* signifies the death-rate at all ages, calculated on the hypothesis that the rate at each of twelve age periods in each town was the same as in England and Wales during the ten years 1871–80, the death-rate at all ages in England and Wales during that period being 21·27 per 1,000.

The *factor for correction* is the figure by which the recorded death-rate should be multiplied in order to correct for variations of sex and age-distribution.

The *corrected death-rate* is the recorded death-rate multiplied by the factor for correction.

The *comparative mortality figure* represents the corrected death-rate in each town, compared with the recorded death-rate, at all ages, in England and Wales, taken as 1,000.

The figures in this column may be read as follows:—After making approximate correction for differences of age and sex-distribution, the same number of living persons that gave 1,000 deaths in England and Wales in 1887 gave 925 in Brighton, 949 in Derby, etc., etc., and 1,701 in Manchester.

The first column in the preceding table is obtained by assuming that the mean mortality in England and Wales in 1871–80 held good in each town. The age and sex-distribution of each town at the last census being known, the mean mortality in England and Wales, 1871–80, is applied to the population thus constituted, and we have as a result the series of death-rates in Col. 1. The differences between the various towns in this column are consequently caused simply and solely by difference in age and sex-distribution. As an example of the method of obtaining these *standard death-rates*, Brighton may be taken.

	Mean Annual Death-rate for England and Wales, 1871–80.		Population of Brighton in 1881.		Calculated number of Deaths.	
Ages.	Males.	Females.	Males.	Females.	Males.	Females.
Under 5	68·14	58·10	6,213	6,371	423·35	370·16
5 to 10	6·67	6·20	5,653	5,533	37·70	34·30
10 to 15	3·69	3·70	5,294	5,447	19·53	20·15
15 to 20	5·23	5·43	4,480	6,512	23·43	35·36
20 to 25	7·32	6·78	4,326	6,398	31·67	43·37
25 to 35	9·30	8·58	7,217	9,927	67·12	85·17
35 to 45	13·74	11·58	5,356	7,305	73·59	84·59
45 to 55	20·05	15·59	3,910	5,552	78·40	86·55
55 to 65	34·76	28·54	2,707	3,988	94·09	113·82
65 to 75	69·57	60·82	1,409	2,343	98·02	142·50
75 and upwards	169·08	155·83	631	974	106·69	151·78
Totals			47,196	60,350	1053·59	1167·75

Here the total population of Brighton in 1881 = 107,546.

The total number of calculated deaths = 2221·34.

The standard death-rate will therefore = 20·66 per 1,000, which corresponds with the rate given in the table on page 92.

Now the annual death-rate of England and Wales in 1871–80 was 21·27. This ought to be the same as the calculated death-rate for Brighton, which has been obtained by applying the mean annual death-rate of England and Wales at the different age-groups to the population of Brighton at these age-groups. But the death-rate for Brighton is *lower*, as shown above, which must arise from the fact that the distribution of age and sex in the Brighton population is more favourable than in the country generally. That this is so will be seen more clearly from the following table, in which the composition of each population per 1,000 is given:—

Age-Distribution of Population. 1881.	At all ages.	0 to 5.	5 to 10.	10 to 15.	15 to 20.	20 to 25.	25 to 35.	35 to 45.	45 to 55.	55 to 65.	65 to 75.	75 and upwards.
England & Wales	1,000	136	120	108	98	90	146	113	83	59	33	14
Brighton . . .	1,000	117	104	100	103	99	159	118	88	62	35	15
Sex-Distribution of same Populations												
Brighton { Males	439	58	53	49	42	40	67	50	36	25	13	6
Brighton { Fem.	561	59	51	51	61	59	92	68	52	37	22	9
England & Wales { Males	486	67	60	54	49	43	70	54	40	28	15	6
England & Wales { Fem.	514	68	61	54	49	47	76	59	43	31	18	8

It is evident that there is a considerably larger proportion of females in the Brighton population, and that while there is a much smaller number of children under 5, there is only a slightly larger proportion of persons over 55, or in other words, at the ages of high mortality.

The standard death-rate being lower for Brighton must be

raised in the same proportion in order to bring it into comparison with the death-rate of England and Wales—*i.e.*, it must be increased in the proportion of 20·66 to 21·27. But the fraction $\frac{21 \cdot 27}{20 \cdot 66} = 1 \cdot 0296$. This, then, is the *factor* for correction for age and sex-distribution by which the recorded death-rate of Brighton must be multiplied in order that it may be comparable with that of England and Wales. It may be objected that the mean age and sex-distribution of the decennium 1871–80 is assumed in the above calculation to hold good for every year of the succeeding decennium. This, however, can be proved to be approximately accurate, inasmuch as in populations whose chief occupations remain the same the age and sex-distribution after a time assumes constant proportions. It may be objected again that the factor or correction figure, which is accurate when applied to the rate of an entire decade, may not be equally accurate for each year of that decade. But on selecting for comparison two years, one extremely hot and therefore dangerous to the young, and the other extremely cold and dangerous to the aged, the Registrar-General found that the error due to the use of the decennial correction figure as a constant, instead of a special correction figure for each year, was so small that it might practically be disregarded.

By multiplying the recorded death-rates in column 3 (page 92) by the factors for correction, we obtain the corrected death-rates given in column 4. These are the death-rates which would have been recorded in each town had its population been identical, so far as age and sex-distribution are concerned, with the population of England and Wales.

Trustworthiness of General Death-Rates.—The following remarks of the Registrar-General (Annual Summary, 1883) on this point are apposite: "It may naturally be asked, of what use are the general death-rates, as usually given, if they cannot be accepted without further and considerable correction? In the first place, if the death-rate in any given town or other area in one year be compared with its death-rates in other years, no correction is required; for the age and sex-distribution in an individual town or other area remains practically constant; and, secondly, although it is doubtlessly true that the general death-rates of towns or other areas cannot safely be used for accurate comparison between such towns or areas in respect of healthiness without further correction, yet they serve as a very valuable approximate indication; for if the column 3 be compared with column 4, it will be seen that whether the towns be arranged according to their recorded or according to their corrected death-rates, the order will scarcely be changed. The correction simply alters the amount of difference between the towns, leaving the position in which they stand to each other but slightly changed."

In the table on page 92 it will be seen that only in two of the twenty-eight towns, Plymouth and Norwich, is the corrected death-rate lower than the recorded death-rate. In all the other towns a correctional addition to the recorded death-rate is required, varying in amount from 0·50 to 3·28.

If the death-rates in the *counties* are corrected for age and sex-distribution, so as to conform to the standard of England and Wales, the corrected rate in the greater number of the counties is somewhat lower than the recorded rate. In the table given at page xviii. of Dr. Ogle's Supplement to the Registrar-General's Report for 1871–80, only ten counties have the corrected rates higher than the recorded rates. Of these ten, all, except the extra-metropolitan parts of Surrey and Middlesex, are industrial counties, where the death-rate even before correction is very high; while all the agricultural counties are comprised in the majority, and have their death-rates, which are already low, lowered by correction. Before correction the extreme limits of variation in the death-rates of different counties lie between 16·77 and 25·17, while after correction they range from 15·97 to 26·87 per 1,000. As a general rule, it may be stated that correction raises the rates of towns and industrial centres, but lowers the rates of rural districts.

Another instance of the importance of correction for age and sex-distribution may be quoted from Dr. Ogle. In 1881 the general death-rate in England and Wales was 18·9 per 1,000 of all ages, while the general death-rate in France was 22·0, *i.e.* 3·1 higher than England. But had the age distribution of the French population been identical with that of the English population, the French general death-rate would have been 20·9 and not 22·0. Thus of the 3·1 difference between the two rates, 2·0 was due to difference of health condition, and 1·1 was due to difference of age distribution.

CHAPTER VII.

MALE AND FEMALE MORTALITY AT DIFFERENT AGES.

Death-Rates at Age-Groups.—False Methods of Estimating these.—Infantile Population.—Infantile Mortality.—Mortality in each Month of First Year.—Causes of Infantile Mortality.—Insurance of Children.—Mortality of Illegitimate Infants.—Female Mortality.—The Standard Million.

IN the last chapter, the disturbing influence of varying age and sex distribution of the population on the general mortality has been discussed, and the method by which the fallacy involved can be avoided has been described. We have also pointed out that the relative position of the twenty-eight great towns is scarcely changed, the correction simply altering the amount of difference between the towns, but leaving their relative position practically the same.

Death-rate at Age-groups.—A statement of the death-rate at various groups of ages per 1,000 living at these ages, is quite trustworthy for comparison with other towns and districts. To obtain this, it is necessary to know—

1. The population at different age-groups.
2. The deaths at different age-groups.

The latter are obtained from the local registrar's death-returns; the former may be ascertained in the case of each urban and rural sanitary authority by an application to each group of ages of the same method of estimation for increase of population as that described on page 6. For the population at all ages the same rate of increase at each group of ages, as in the previous intercensal period, is assumed to continue during the present decennium. Thus, if the numbers living at each age-group in 1871 and 1881 are known from the census returns, the calculation is short. If, however, in the 1871 census, the age-constitution of the population in question was not given, a subsidiary calculation is required. It is assumed that the age-distribution does not vary between the two census enumerations, an assumption practically correct when the prevailing industry in a given neighbourhood has not altered. Then having given the total population in 1881 and in 1871, and the population distributed according to age and sex in 1881, the finding of the distributed population of 1886 is a mere question of proportion.

Thus if the total population of a town in 1881 is 107,546, and the number living aged 10–15 is 10,741, while the total population in 1871 is 92,481, to find the number living aged 10–15 in 1886.

The calculation will be in three stages.

(1) Find rate of increase per unit of population from 1871 to 1881.

$$92481(1+r)^{10}=107546.$$

$$\text{Therefore } 1+r=\sqrt[10]{\frac{107546}{92481}}.$$

$$\text{And log. }(1+r)=\tfrac{1}{10}\text{ (log. }107546-\text{log. }92481).$$

$$\text{Therefore } 1+r=1{\cdot}015.$$

And r=rate of increase per unit of population=·015.

(2) Find from this the total mean population for 1886, *i.e.* after the lapse of $5\frac{1}{4}$ years. If P=mean population of 1886.

$$P=107546\ (1{\cdot}015)^{\frac{21}{4}}.$$

$$\text{Hence } P=116363.$$

(3) Find in this population the number living aged 10–15.

If x=this number,

Then $107546 : 116363 :: 10741 : x$.

Therefore $x=\underline{11625}$.

There are *two false methods* of estimating the rate of mortality at different ages. The first of these is to calculate the proportion of deaths to total deaths; and the second to calculate the proportion of deaths at various age-groups to the population at all ages. The fallacy involved in the first method arises from the fact that either a diminution in the total deaths or an increase in the deaths at any age-group would increase the proportional deaths at the age-group under consideration, though its interpretation in the two cases would be essentially different. Or if a reduction in both the total deaths and the deaths at a given age-group occurred, this reduction might be entirely hidden by the statement of the result as a proportion between the two.

The second method is equally fallacious; as apart from any conditions adverse to health, the number of deaths at various age-groups, and therefore the proportion of these to the entire population, will vary with the number living at the same age-groups.

For *small populations* a too minute division of age-groups is unadvisable. Deductions from a small number of individual facts are never so trustworthy as when the basis on which an inference is founded is wider, and accidental causes of variation are thus to a large extent eliminated.

The following table gives the death-rates at various age-groups per 1,000 living at these age-groups.

It will be seen that under 5 and over 55 the death-rate per 1,000 living at each group of ages is higher than the general death-rate at all ages; while at intermediate ages the mortality is lower than the general death-rate, being at its lowest ebb between 10 and 15, and much lower between 5 and 25 than at succeeding ages. It is evident, therefore, that the age-distribution which would be most favourable to a low mortality is one containing an undue proportion of persons aged 5 to 25—such a population as would naturally arise from a continuously high birth-rate.

Annual Death-rates in England and Wales at Twelve Groups of Ages in Groups of Years, 1838-87.*—*Males and Females.*

PERIOD.	AGES.												
	All Ages.	0-	5-	10-	15-	20-	25-	35-	45-	55-	65-	75-	85 and upwds.
	DEATHS TO 1,000 LIVING.												
	MALES.												
1838 to 1886	**22·8**	**70·1**	**7·9**	**4·4**	**6·2**	**8·3**	**9·5**	**13·1**	**18·9**	**32·8**	**67·6**	**147·7**	**313·5**
1838–40	23·3	72·6	9·7	5·3	7·3	9·5	10·2	12·9	18·2	32·1	65·8	144·0	306·2
1841–50	23·1	71·2	9·2	5·1	7·1	9·5	9·9	12·9	18·2	31·8	67·5	148·3	312·3
1851–60	23·1	72·7	8·5	4·9	6·7	8·8	9·6	12·5	18·0	31·0	65·5	146·7	308·2
1861–70	23·7	73·5	8·2	4·5	6·2	8·5	9·9	13·5	19·2	33·1	67·1	147·2	315·0
1871–80	22·7	68·5	6·7	3·7	5·3	7·4	9·4	13·8	20·1	34·9	69·7	150·8	327·4
1881–85	20·4	59·6	5·8	3·2	4·6	6·0	8·2	12·7	19·4	33·6	68·8	144·6	296·4
1886	20·3	60·3	4·6	2·8	4·3	5·6	7·6	12·0	19·3	33·5	72·7	151·0	333·0
1887	19·8	57·8	4·9	2·9	4·2	5·3	7·4	11·9	18·8	33·5	72·0	146·7	303·5
	FEMALES.												
1838 to 1886	**20·8**	**60·3**	**7·7**	**4·6**	**6·7**	**7·9**	**9·5**	**12·1**	**15·6**	**28·0**	**59·8**	**134·3**	**288·1**
1838–40	21·5	62·4	9·4	5·8	8·3	9·1	10·3	12·7	15·8	28·1	57·3	130·0	278·4
1841–50	21·6	61·1	8·9	5·4	7·9	9·1	10·6	12·9	16·1	28·4	60·9	135·9	293·3
1851–60	21·4	63·0	8·4	5·1	7·4	8·6	10·0	12·2	15·3	27·1	58·9	134·5	288·9
1861–70	21·4	63·7	7·8	4·5	6·7	8·0	9·7	12·1	15·6	27·9	59·1	134·9	285·1
1871–80	20·1	58·4	6·3	3·7	5·5	6·8	8·6	11·6	15·6	28·7	61·0	135·4	296·4
1881–85	18·2	50·5	5·6	3·3	4·7	5·9	7·9	10·9	15·2	27·8	59·5	129·4	267·8
1886	18·3	50·9	4·7	3·1	4·5	5·3	7·2	10·3	15·0	28·4	64·2	137·6	307·0
1887	17·8	48·9	4·9	3·0	4·3	5·5	7·1	10·2	15·2	28·0	63·4	132·7	276·2

It has often been asked why, in a population with a continuously high birth-rate, these inequalities in the proportion of persons living at the different groups of ages do not in a series of years adjust themselves. This cannot be answered better than in Mr. N. A. Humphreys' words: "It must be

* The populations used are deduced from the rates of increase observed in the 40 years 1841-81, and are distributed in the several groups of ages according to the proportions found to prevail at the last five censuses.

CHART OF DEATH RATES
AT DIFFERENT AGE-GROUPS. 1886.

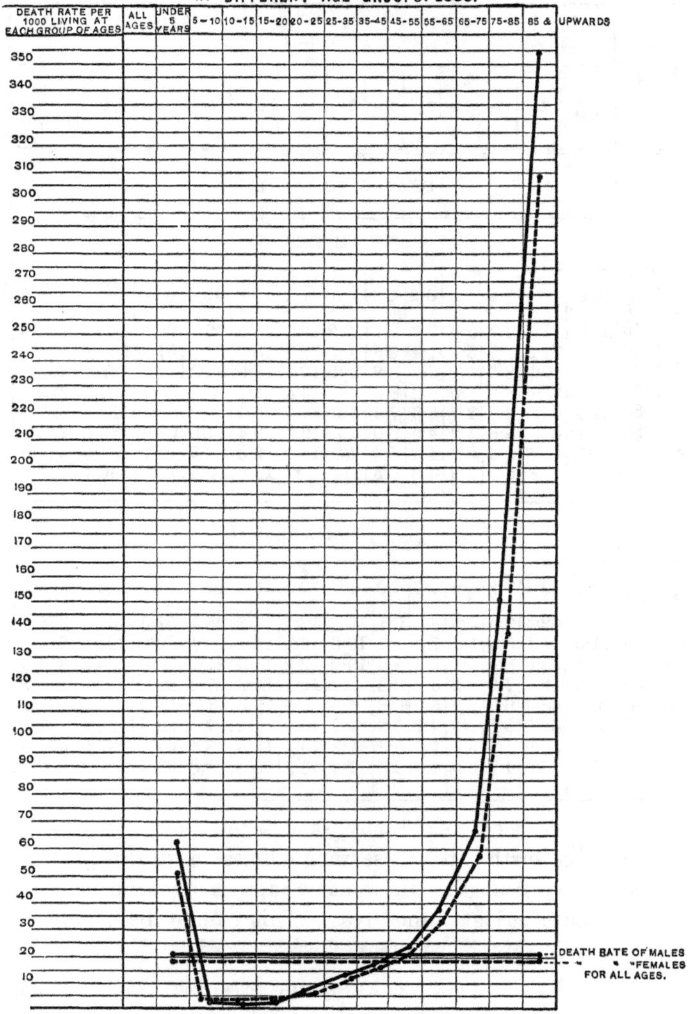

remembered that an annually increasing number of births forms a continuously recurring wave, which is always raising the proportion of those living at the lower ages, and which cannot cease its disturbing influence unless the birth-rate were for a lengthened period to remain stationary, as is assumed in a Life-Table population."

Infantile Population.—In considering the mortality at different ages, the first group of ages (under 5) requires further consideration, and especially the mortality under one year of age (infantile mortality). In order to ascertain the infantile mortality, it is necessary to know the infantile population. And in this case the census enumerations do not give us information which is as trustworthy as in most cases. The ages of infants are very commonly incorrectly returned at the census. The number under one year old is certainly understated (many in their first year being returned as one year old). A smaller number in their second year are returned as two years old, and so on. It has been sought to explain the deficiency of infants returned at the census by omissions in enumeration, but Dr. Farr has attributed it rightly to confusion between the current year of age and the completed years of life, rather than to actual omissions. On account of this deficiency in the census number of infants, it is more trustworthy to estimate their *mortality in proportion to every thousand births.* A more strictly correct plan would be to take the mean of the births of the current and the immediately preceding year as giving the true infantile population; but as this plan is not usually adopted, for the sake of uniformity the births of the current year are taken.

Infantile Mortality.—The infantile mortality then is the annual number of deaths of infants under one year of age to every thousand births during the same year. Dr. Rumsey regarded the infantile mortality as a most reliable test, owing to the fact that migration does not greatly affect the result at this early age. He held, however, that premature births should be struck out of account both of the living and dying. It should be remembered that still-births are in this country thus excluded from registration, though in France they are included. Probably the best plan would be to insist on registration in every case, making a class separate from births and deaths, in which still-births and premature births would find a logical place.

A table showing the infantile mortality in the different counties of England and Wales is given at page 58. This table shows that the infantile mortality is usually lowest in agricultural neighbourhoods and highest in industrial centres. The following table compares the infantile mortality of the 28 great towns during 1887 :—

Towns.	*Deaths under One Year to 1,000 Births.*	
	Ten Years, 1877-86.	1887.
England and Wales . .	142	145
28 Towns	161	168
London	152	158
Brighton	148	149
Portsmouth	138	143
Norwich	173	158
Plymouth	157	196
Bristol	145	149
Wolverhampton . . .	159	176
Birmingham	164	176
Leicester	201	209
Nottingham	175	170
Derby	143	142
Birkenhead	137	156
Liverpool	183	186
Bolton	177	171
Manchester	174	191
Salford	178	195
Oldham	169	187
Blackburn	187	201
Preston	218	214
Huddersfield	169	181
Halifax	159	153
Bradford	162	178
Leeds	172	172
Sheffield	163	177
Hull	161	165
Sunderland	157	151
Newcastle	160	174
Cardiff	169	172

Mortality of Infants in each Month of First Year.—Life is most liable to perish in its earliest stages, "the liability decreasing in something like geometrical progression until the body becomes developed and the reproductive function is established, when the chances of destruction again increase, the succession of the species being thus secured" (Rumsey). With each week after birth the danger of death diminishes. For this reason it is advisable in dealing with large populations to state the monthly or even weekly mortality of infants. The rate of mortality of boys in every month of the first year of life exceeds that of girls, so that, spite of the much larger number of boys at birth, they do not greatly exceed the number of girls at the end of the first year. The following table from the Registrar-General's 38th Annual Report (1875) gives the annual rate of mortality per 1,000 living at each month of age:—

Annual Death-Rate per 1,000 at each Month of Age.

Age in Months.	In Healthy Districts.	By English Life Table.	In Liverpool District.
0	447·51	571·32	672·19
1	145·49	218·37	316·72
2	102·05	157·10	226·78
3	87·16	131·87	209·37
4	81·09	126·04	205·25
5	75·54	120·50	203·65
6	70·54	115·09	204·89
7	65·97	109·92	209·17
8	61·85	105·01	216·42
9	58·32	100·33	227·30
10	55·28	95·84	241·80
11	52·86	91·61	260·23

It will be seen that the conditions of life in a large town like Liverpool are so unfavourable to infantile life, that the mortality is in some months double that in the healthy districts, while at the seventh month and upwards it is more than three times as great.

Causes of Infantile Mortality.—Some of the causes of infantile mortality are common to every locality. Such are—

(1) *Prematurity of birth* and *congenital defects.* The health conditions under which the mother lives have an undoubted influence on the vitality of her progeny, and on the occurrence of premature birth.

(2) *Hereditary tendencies*, such as the inheritance of syphilis, or degradation and drunkenness of parents, have also a very important influence. Dr. Hope has suggested some check on the marriage of unsuitable people, securing the greatest good of the greatest number, and, in Dr. Farr's words, rendering "growth more perfect, decay less rapid, life more vigorous, and death more remote."

(3) The inexperience and *neglect of mothers*, especially of the industrial classes, is a most important factor in infantile mortality. As regards *inexperience*, it has been suggested that the deaths of first-born children should be separated from the general infantile mortality. Such returns would undoubtedly show that first-born children die at a higher rate than children of a later birth; but some of the excess would be attributable to greater difficulty in parturition, as well as to parental inexperience. In the year 1875 the mean infantile mortality in twelve urban districts, which Dr. Farr tabulated, was 192 per 1,000 births, and the mean proportion of women who *married under* 21 to every 100 marriages was 28; whereas in twelve rural districts, in which the mean infantile mortality was 92 per 1,000 births, the percentage of marriages of minors was only 18. Neglect on the part of parents is largely due to—

(4) *Industrial conditions.* In the large centres of industry the employment of women in mills during pregnancy and at an early interval after childbirth has a most deleterious effect on the welfare of their infants. The latter are sent out to nurse during the day, and commonly fed on farinaceous food instead of milk, which constitutes the natural food of infancy. It has been suggested that the employment of women in mills, etc., should not be allowed for one year after childbirth, and that the local registrar should have instructions to furnish when

each birth is registered simple printed directions concerning the food and general management of infants. Dr. Ashby estimates that among the working classes in large manufacturing towns the number of deaths under one year of age is equal to one-third of the number under five, and represents about one-half of the total deaths at all ages.

(5) *Improper food* and methods of feeding are responsible for a large share of infantile mortality. The improper substitution of farinaceous for milk food has been already mentioned. The use of uncleanly bottles containing milk in an incipient state of putrefaction is a common source of infantile diarrhœa. The close connection between methods of feeding and infantile mortality is shown by the fact that during the sufferings and starvation connected with the siege of Paris in 1870–71, while the general mortality was doubled, that of infants is said to have been reduced by about 40 per cent., owing to mothers being obliged to suckle their infants. The same increase of adult and diminution of infant mortality was seen during the Lancashire cotton famine, when mothers were not at work at the mills. When improper feeding is a chief factor in producing infantile mortality, then a large proportion of the deaths are from diarrhœa and digestive diseases. Convulsions, again, are very commonly due to the irritation produced by improper food. The administration of opiates in the form of "soothing syrups," etc., and the dosing of children with medicines of various kinds, apart from medical advice, constitute another cause of much evil. On the other hand, the neglect to obtain early medical attendance in illness not uncommonly leads to fatal consequences.

(6) The deaths from accidental or homicidal *violence* require consideration. In 1886 nearly half the total murders—81 out of 171—were cases of infanticide, *i.e.* murders of children in the first year and generally the first month of life; and more than 10 per cent. of the deaths ascribed to manslaughter were also deaths of infants. Taking these two together, the mean annual death-rate from homicide during the years 1858–86 was 183 for males, and 189 for females, per million births of each sex.

Among the industrial classes, death is occasionally due to

suffocation from *overlaying* of infants. It has been repeatedly noted that such deaths are especially common on Saturday nights and holidays, and there is little doubt that they are frequently due to the drunkenness of parents.

(7) *Insurance of infants*, ostensibly to provide funeral expenses in case of death, to say the least, constitutes an additional hazard for the children. This is practically acknowledged by the Insurance Offices doing this kind of business, in the rates of premium they charge, which are enormously in excess of what would be required to cover actual risks, as shown by the English Life Table. £6 is the legal limit of insurance for a child under five; but the fact that in such cases parents have a direct pecuniary interest in the death of their children is found to lead to a much greater rate of mortality among insured than among uninsured children.

If the general mortality of the great towns (p. 85) be compared with their infantile mortality (p. 104), it will be seen that there is not necessarily a close association between the two. The infantile mortality is largely governed by the amount of summer diarrhœa (p. 189), but the origin of the excessive amount of this and of infantile mortality from all causes in some towns requires further elucidation.

Effect of Illegitimacy on Infantile Mortality.—An examination of the table on p. 58 does not show any constant relation between the rate of illegitimacy and the entire infantile mortality. Possibly a certain number of illegitimate births are in towns registered as legitimate, while in rural districts they are correctly registered; some illegitimate children again escape registration altogether. If, however, we separate the births of legitimate and illegitimate children, and adopt a like method for the corresponding deaths, a very different result is obtained. Thus, in the years 1871–75, the mean mortality of infants in twelve urban districts was, for legitimate children, 192 per 1,000 legitimate births; for illegitimate children, 388 per 1,000 illegitimate births. In Glasgow, during 1873–75, the annual deaths of legitimate infants to every 1,000 legitimate births were 152; of illegitimate infants to every 1,000 illegitimate births, 286. The following more recent figures from Dr. Tatham's Annual Report for 1887 may be compared with the preceding statistics.

Births and Deaths of Illegitimate Infants in Salford.

Years.	Births.		Percentage of Illegitimate Births to Total Births.	Deaths Under One Year.		Proportion of Deaths Under One Year per 1,000 Births.		
	Total.	Illegit.		Total.	Illegit.	Total.	Legit.	Illegit.
1887 . . .	6,956	321	4·6	1,357	119	195	187	371
Eight years, 1879–86 .	56,492	2,506	4·4	10,127	918	179	171	366

In the face of such facts, the importance of illegitimacy as a national calamity is evident, and the following remarks, quoted by Dr. Farr from Von Bernoulli, are so apposite that we reproduce them here: "The invariable fact that the mortality among the illegitimate is far greater than among the legitimate, and that many more of them are still-born, shows clearly enough how much more unfavourable their position is from the first. Who can doubt that their bringing up is much harder and more difficult?—that the existence of a class of men, bound to society by few or no family ties, is not a matter of indifference to the State? The great majority of foundlings are illegitimate, which of itself shows how little, as a general rule, the mothers can or will care for these children. It is beyond doubt that fewer illegitimate children grow up to maturity,—that they get through the world with more trouble, than children born in wedlock,—that more of them are poor, and that therefore more of them become criminals. Illegitimacy is in itself an evil to a man; and the State should seek to diminish the number of these births, and carefully inquire to what circumstances any increase is to be ascribed."

The following table gives the deaths of infants in England

and Wales during 1887 from various causes, and in a parallel column the total deaths during the same period:—

Infantile and Total Deaths in 1887.

Causes of Death.	Under One Year.		At All Ages.	
	Males.	Females.	Males.	Females.
From All Causes	71,463	56,814	272,137	258,621
Measles	1,902	1,485	8,657	8,108
Scarlet Fever	239	205	3,899	3,960
Diphtheria	134	91	2,116	2,327
Whooping Cough	2,195	2,555	4,928	6,623
Diarrhœa	7,750	6,351	10,725	9,517
Parasitic Diseases	362	278	445	379
Dietetic Diseases	145	124	1,099	666
Constitutional Diseases	4,713	3,537	44,181	45,223
Developmental Diseases	9,479	7,355	21,219	22,714
Local Diseases	30,611	23,241	140,761	133,776
Violence	1,091	1,044	12,979	5,146
Ill-Defined and not Specified	11,389	9,279	14,578	12,387

Death-rate at other Age-Groups.—Of these the one requiring special mention is the *death-rate* of children *under* 5 *years old*, which, like all other rates, should be calculated on the number of children living at these ages. This forms, perhaps, a more important sanitary test than the death-rate at any subsequent age-period. By the English Life Table, No. 3, of 1,000 children born, 150 die in the first year, 54 in the second, 28 in the third, 18 in the fourth, and 14 in the fifth year of life, making a total of 264 deaths in the first five years of life. Of the 150 who die in the first year of life, 50 die in the first month, and 20 in the second. The tables on pages 88 and 101 give the death-rate under 5 for different periods, and it will be seen that there has been a considerable gain at these earlier periods, while at the higher age-groups there is a slight increase of mortality.

Dr. Farr has adopted a quinquennial grouping of ages before 25, and after this age a decennial, odd figures being selected as the limiting ages of the groups (25–35, etc.). This method was adopted in order to avoid the fallacy caused by the tendency which both the census and death-returns showed to state ages at round figures as 20, 30, etc. It might be supposed that smaller groups of years would give more valuable results; but it must be remembered that the age-distribution of the population and the ages registered at death are not yet entirely trustworthy, and that the elaboration of groups would tend to diminish the true value of the results obtained. Dr. Farr states the case against further differentiation of groups thus: "In exhibiting such an abstract, I should commit a fault which I deem it most important to avoid—that of assuming the delusive appearance of more minute accuracy than actually exists."

Dr. Ransome has suggested that inasmuch as the general death-rate is open to criticism as a test of sanitary condition, the *death-rate under the age of* 15 should be employed. He points out that "few comparatively leave their homes under 15 years; consequently, up to this period of life, the population of any particular place may be looked upon as tolerably stationary." This is probably true of Manchester, to which the remarks particularly apply, but in many towns there is considerable migration to boarding schools, etc. In addition, this test is defective, as it relates only to a small part of life, leaving out of consideration the ages between 15 and 55, when persons are of an age and strength for remunerative labour. On the whole, we should prefer the general death-rate to this, though the two in conjunction would give more reliable indications of sanitary status than either alone; and better still is the death-rate at the different age-groups given by the Registrar-General. For small populations, however, the age-groups selected should not be too small, as the trustworthiness of death-rates diminishes steadily with the decrease of the number of facts on which the rates are founded.

A recent address by Mr. Chadwick to the Association of Sanitary Inspectors (August, 1888), forms an illustration of an important fallacy. He stated that in Brighton the deaths of children under 5 years of age formed 35·17 per cent., while among the rich they were only 8·9 per cent. of the total deaths

Death-Rate at all Ages of Males and Females.

Years.	Males.	Females.
1838–40	23·3	21·5
1841–50	23·1	21·6
1851–60	23·1	21·4
1861–70	23·7	21·4
1871–80	22·7	20·1
1881–85	20·4	18·2
1886	20·3	18·3
1887	19·8	17·8

It might be inferred that inasmuch as (*a*) the proportionate number of males with their higher rate of mortality is diminishing in the population, and (*b*) the female death-rate is decreasing more rapidly than the male, the recent improvement in general mortality is due to these causes, and not to an improvement of the condition under which the male population lives. Mr. Humphreys has shown, however, that the disturbing influence of sex-distribution on the general death-rate is but slight. As determined by the English Life-Table, the male mortality is 25·05, and the female mortality 23·90 per 1,000. Thus if it were possible to have two different populations, consisting of males and females separately, the death-rate of the male population would exceed that of the female population by 1·15 per 1,000, on the assumption that sanitary conditions were equal, and the age-distribution of the two populations was normal. This represents the greatest possible error, and such an extreme case is impossible. The excess of female population actually present in any district has so small an influence that it may be practically neglected.

In his 50th Annual Report (for 1887), the Registrar-General has pointed out that the ordinary method of giving the death-rates of males and females—that is to give the proportion of annual deaths to a million or a thousand living of each sex—is faulty for purposes of strict comparison, owing to the fact that the age distribution differs greatly in the two sexes. Thus among females there is a much larger proportion of very aged persons and a much smaller proportion of very young children than among males in the general population, and the mortality from any disease which specially affects infancy would be unfairly lowered in the case of women, the reverse holding good for the diseases of old age. The only mode of making a fair comparison between the sexes is to calculate, by means of the rates at the successive age-periods, the mortality in a million, in which the age-distribution is the same for each sex. This million is termed by the Registrar-General *a standard million*, and is a million with the age-distribution of the general population of England and Wales at the date of the 1881 census, as shown in the following table:—

Age.	Proportion per Million.	Age.	Proportion per Million.
All Ages	1,000,000	25–35	146,048
Under 5	135,551	35–45	113,217
5–10	121,172	45–55	83,676
10–15	107,811	55–65	59,062
15–20	98,067	65–75	32,818
20–25	89,635	75 and upwards	12,943

The *causes of the higher mortality among men* are largely connected with the greater hardships and dangers of their occupations. These will be fully discussed in Chapter IX. The greater amount of intemperance among men has no inconsiderable influence in the same direction.

CHAPTER VIII.

INFLUENCE OF CLIMATIC AND SOCIAL CONDITIONS ON MORTALITY.

Influence of Climate.—Influence of Season.—Mild Winters and Cool Summers.—Seasonal Prevalence of Diseases.—Cyclical Changes.—Effect of Conditions of Subsoil.—Effect of Race.—Effect of Marital Condition.—Effect of Sanitation.—Increased Urban Population and lowered Mortality.—Effect of Sanitation on Phthisis and Typhoid Fever.—School Life and Mortality.

WE have in the two last chapters discussed the effect of varying age and sex distribution on the general death-rate, and the death-rate at different age-groups. Before considering the mortality from special diseases, the influence of climatic and social conditions, of density of population, and occupation require attention, and to these the present and two subsequent chapters will be devoted.

The influence of climate cannot easily be separated from that of other conditions of environment. To obtain trustworthy statistics under this head, it would be necessary to eliminate the effect of variations in the age distribution of the populations compared, of density of population, staple industries, and of differences in food and in other particulars. Thus the Army Reports for different foreign and home stations, which would appear a most promising field of investigation in this connection, not only exhibit the influence of climate, but also of the sanitary condition of barracks, etc. It would be well in investigations concerning climate to consider separately its effect on strangers and on the indigenous inhabitants.

Season has an influence which can be stated in figures. As shown in the following table, in five out of the six years,

1881–6, the general mortality is highest in the first quarter of the year, and lowest in the third quarter. This low mortality in the third quarter of the year would be still more marked but for the prevalence of Summer Diarrhœa.

Town and Country Districts of England and Wales.—Annual Death-Rates in each Quarter of the Six Years, 1881–86.

	Area in Acres.	Estimated Population in the middle of 1886.	Quarter ending.	Annual Rate of Mortality per 1,000 in each quarter of the Years 1881.	1882.	1883.	1884.	1885.	1886.
England and Wales . . .	37,239,351	27,870,586	Year .	**18·9**	**19·6**	**19·5**	**19·5**	**19·0**	**19·3**
			March	21·5	21·5	22·2	19·5	21·8	22·8
			June .	18·6	19·0	20 0	18·9	19·3	18·0
			Sept. .	16·8	17·8	16·8	19·7	16·5	17·8
			Dec. .	18·7	20·0	19·2	19·9	18·5	18·5
Town Districts. All Registration Sub-Districts three-fourths of the population of which, as enumerated in 1881, resided within the boundaries of Urban Sanitary Districts existing in 1886	3,688,436	17,716,932	Year .	**20·1**	**20·9**	**20·5**	**20·6**	**19·7**	**20·0**
			March	22·6	22·9	23·0	20·3	22·1	23·3
			June .	19·2	20·0	20·6	19·6	20·0	18·2
			Sept. .	18·3	19·3	18·1	21·5	17·5	19·1
			Dec. .	20·2	21·4	20·5	21·0	19·4	19·4
Country Districts. All the remaining Registration Sub-Districts of England and Wales, — not coming within the above definition of Town Districts	33,550,915	10,153,654	Year .	**16·9**	**17·3**	**17·9**	**17·7**	**17·8**	**18·0**
			March	19·7	19·2	21·0	18·3	21·3	22·0
			June .	17·5	17·4	19·2	17·7	18·2	17·7
			Sept. .	14·2	15·2	14·6	16·7	14·7	15·6
			Dec. .	16·1	17·6	16·9	18·0	17·1	16 8

Dr. Edward Smith's elaborate physiological researches have

a bearing on seasonal mortality. He found that the amount of carbonic acid eliminated was much greater in winter than in summer. Corresponding with these facts, Mr. Milner, the medical superintendent of the Wakefield prison, found that the prisoners uniformly lost weight during the first and fourth quarters of the year, and gained weight during the second and third quarters, the gain beginning about the end of March, and the loss at the beginning of September, about the same time as Dr. Smith found a similar change in the amount of carbonic acid eliminated.

The effect of season appears to be more than can be explained by the physical phenomena of temperature and atmospheric pressure. Even with the same amount of exertion, less carbonic acid is apparently evolved in summer than in winter, as compared with the corresponding amounts when at rest at these two periods. These facts have important bearings on the viability of children born at different seasons of the year, Dr. E. Smith concluding that the viability is greatest for children born in the winter or spring months. Other factors are doubtless also at work.

Mild winters and cool summers both lower the mortality, the former especially of the old, and the latter of the young, and especially of the infantile population. A cold, damp summer is always accompanied by a low mortality. During the third quarter of 1887 the death-rate in England and Wales was 3·0 per 1,000 below the mean rate in the corresponding periods of the ten years 1878–87, and considerably lower than that recorded in the third quarter of any year since the beginning of civil registration in 1837. The mean temperature of the quarter was 57·6° Fahr., or 2·1° below the average for the corresponding quarters of 117 years. The amount of rain at Greenwich was 11·21 inches, or 3·93 inches above the average amount in corresponding periods of 73 years. The number of hours of sunshine recorded at the Royal Observatory was 361·5, or 81·3 hours below the average amount of the ten years 1878–87.

Season has also an important influence on the character of

prevalent diseases, intestinal diseases being most prevalent in summer, and respiratory diseases in winter.

Seasonal Prevalence of Diseases.—The following table from Netten Radcliffe's article in Quain's Dictionary of Medicine, shows the seasonal prevalence of various diseases and causes of death.

	Winter.			Spring.			Summer.			Autumn.		
	Jan.	Feb.	Mar.	Apr.	May.	June.	July.	Aug.	Sept.	Oct.	Nov.	Dec.
Small-Pox . . .	+	+	+	+	‡	+	−	−	=	−	−	−
Measles	+	−	−	−	+	‡	+	−	−	−	+	‡
Scarlet Fever . . .	−	−	−	−	−	−	−	+	+	‡	+	+
Diphtheria	+	+	−	−	−	−	−	−	+	+	‡	‡
Whooping Cough . .	+	+	+	+	+	−	−	=	=	=	−	+
Typhus (6 years) . .	+	+	+	+	−	−	+	−	−	+	−	+
Typhoid (6 years) . .	+	+	−	−	−	=	−	+	+	+	‡	+
Erysipelas	+	+	−	−	−	−	−	−	−	+	‡	‡
Diarrhœa and Cholera	−	−	−	−	−	−	‡	‡	+	−	−	−
Old Age	‡	+	+	+	−	−	=	−	−	−	−	+

+ Above average. − Below average. ‡ Maxima. = Minima.

It will be seen from this table that *Enteric Fever* is least prevalent in late spring and early summer, and most prevalent in the autumn. Dr. Longstaff's researches show that, according to the statistics of the London Fever Hospital, the minimum is in April, and the maximum in October. According to the Metropolitan Asylums Board Hospitals returns combined with the returns of deaths in London since 1869, there is a June and July minimum with a more rapid rise to a maximum about the end of October or beginning of November. In all cases the mean is reached about the end of the year, and then occurs a gradual fall to a minimum in April, sometimes interrupted by a slight outbreak in January or February. The curve of *Scarlet Fever* is very similar to that of enteric fever, but its minimum is in March, and it rises more gradually to a maximum in the first week of November. For *Typhus Fever* the prevalence in London, as indicated by the mortality and number of admissions to hospitals, shows a minimum in July, August, or September, rising to a maximum in October, or more usually November; and usually continuing excessive during the winter, with another maximum in January or February, commonly higher than the autumn maximum. Its prevalence may decline suddenly to a minimum in March, or more gradually, the minimum being reached as late as May.

Seasonal Curve of Typhoid Fever.

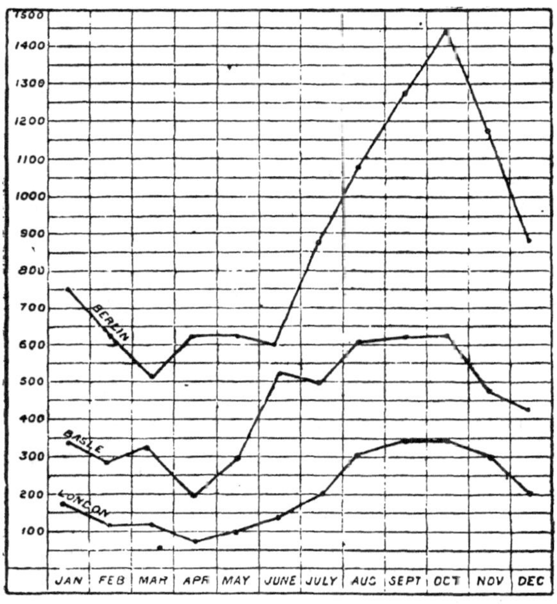

[NOTE.—*The Berlin curve represents the time of death of the patients; those of Basle and London the time of their reception into hospital.*]

Cyclical Changes.—The fact that certain diseases, especially those of an infectious character, recur after an interval of years, shows that, apart from the influence of the season of year, there are periods of change which require for their completion a series of years. Mr. Netten Radcliffe has drawn attention to the fact that the law of periodicity of epidemic and pandemic diseases is not yet determined. Two factors appear to be at work: (1) the influence of an accumulation of susceptible persons in the intervals between two epidemics of the same disease; and (2) certain extraneous conditions which appear to be operative in determining the periodicity, but about which little or nothing is known. The first factor is exemplified by the fluctuations in the amount of small-pox in England, which have been observed to have a close relationship with the fluctuations in the number of unvaccinated children,—a relationship so close that the periods of recurrence of epidemic small-pox could be pretty accurately forecasted. The second factor appears to be exemplified by the fact that, in 1871, when one of the periods of epidemic increase was due, some other undetermined condition gave to the epidemic of 1871–72 a severe character not observed in small-pox since the general introduction of vaccination. Mr. Radcliffe gives as other instances of a similar character the great epidemic of syphilis in the fifteenth century; the exceptional development of fatal diarrhœa in this century; the great development of diphtheria within the last thirty years; and the appearance within recent years of cerebro-spinal fever; which he regards as evidences of secular-pathological changes, to which a clue must be sought by studying their relation with secular meteorological and telluric changes. The solution of the problem why cholera is now endemic in India, then becomes epidemic, and finally pandemic at intervals, belongs to the same category.

Effect of Conditions of Subsoil.—It is well known that respiratory diseases are more prevalent in districts with a cold, damp soil than elsewhere, and that diphtheria and rheumatism also prevail to a greater extent in such districts. The table on p. 129 shows the diminution in mortality from phthisis and typhoid fever which has followed on the execution of main drainage works, which among other things have tended to drain and dry the subsoil. The following statistics tend to throw some doubt on the essential cause of the diminution in the prevalence of phthisis. It will be observed that in West Sussex, which is chiefly an agricultural district, and in which no main drainage is to any great extent in use, phthisis does not vary in amount as the soil becomes more or less pervious to moisture, though lung diseases and diphtheria do so in a striking manner. The figures are derived from Dr. C. Kelly's Annual Report on the Health of West Sussex, a district which covers an area of 335,492 square acres, or about 524 square miles, with a population in 1887 of 105,520. The different soils found in this district are (1) pervious soils, which include the upper and lower greensands, the chalk and the lower Tunbridge Wells sands; (2) the retentive soils, which include the Weald clay, the clayey beds of the lower greensand and the gault; and (3) moderately pervious soils, sloping from the sea to the South Downs, where the chalk is covered for a depth of 15 to 50 feet with loam and brick-earth.

Nature of Soil.	Population.	Death-Rate per 1,000,000 Living at all Ages from			
		Phthisis.	Lung Disease.	Diphtheria.	All Causes.
Pervious . . .	33,820	1514	2131	127	14,852
Moderately Pervious .	29,640	1467	1892	216	14,463
Retentive . .	23,530	1542	2583	454	14,942
West Sussex .	86,990	1506	2172	246	14,741

These figures show that the mortality from diphtheria and lung diseases is much higher on retentive than on pervious soils, while that from phthisis and from all causes is very nearly the same on each variety of soil.

Another table given by Dr. Kelly shows that West Sussex has participated in the great decrease in mortality from phthisis which is to be noticed throughout England, but that this decrease is not confined to the districts with pervious soil, or apparently greater in them than in the districts with retentive soil.

Effect of Race.—The following table shows the death-rate in different countries; but it is obvious that other causes of difference are at work in addition to race.

Death-Rates per 1,000 *Living in Different Countries.*

Countries.	Mean Annual Death-Rate in the 20 years, 1861–80.	1881.	1882.	1883.	1884.	1885.	1886.	1887.
England & Wales	21·9	18·9	19·6	19·5	19·5	19·0	19·3	18·8
Scotland . . .	21·9	19·3	19·3	20·1	19·4	19·1	18·6	18·7
Ireland. . . .	17·5 (17 yrs.)	17·5	17·4	19·2	17·6	18·4	17·9	18·3
Denmark . . .	19·7	18·3	19·3	18·4	18·4	17·9	18·2	18·3
Norway . . .	16·9 (10 yrs.)	16·8	16·4	17·1	16·4	16·5	16·1	—
Sweden . . .	19·2	17·7	17·4	17·3	17·5	17·8	16·6	—
Austria. . . .	31·1	30·6	30·8	30·1	29·2	29·9	29·4	28·9
Hungary . . .	38·7 (15 yrs.)	35·6	36·6	32·6	31·4	—	32·2	—
Switzerland . .	23·6 (11 yrs.)	22·4	21·9	20·3	20·1	21·1	20·4	—
German Empire .	26·9 (9 yrs.)	25·5	25·7	25·9	26·0	25·7	26·2	24·2
Netherlands . .	24·7	21·5	20·7	21·8	22·2	21·0	21·8	19·7
Belgium . . .	22·8	20·9	20·2	20·8	20·9	20·1	21·1	19·3
France	23·6	22·0	22·2	22·2	22·2	21·9	22·5	20·0
Italy	30·0 (18 yrs.)	27·6	27·5	27·5	26·7	26·6	28·3	27·7

The United States would appear to be the best field for this inquiry, as its population is largely recruited by immigration. The following figures are given rather as exemplifying the difficulties of the problem than as justifying a definite conclusion. In 1870, according to Buck, 14·4 per cent. of its aggregate population consisted of foreign-born; viz., Irish, 4·8 per cent.; Germans, 4·4 per cent.; English and Welsh, 1·6 per cent.; all other nationalities (none over 1 per cent.) amounting together to 3·6 per cent. In the same year the population of New York consisted of 45 per cent. foreign-born, of whom 21·4 per cent. were Irish. In 1875, by the State census, 34·2 per cent. of the Boston population consisted of foreigners. But, although the deaths among these different races are separately stated, anomalous age distribution makes it very difficult to institute comparisons. The general death-rates are of no value for this purpose. General Walker has attempted to show that the different foreign populations are similarly constituted as to age, and can therefore be compared amongst themselves. But we refrain from quoting his figures, as it is probable that social conditions and overcrowding (especially among the Irish) are more potent in producing the differences observed than race.

Dr. Beddoe, in his article on "Mortality" in Quain's Dictionary of Medicine, gives the Jews as the best example of the influence of race apart from habits of life; as, for instance, at Frankfort-on-Maine, where the mean age at death of Christians is stated to be 36·9 years, of Jews, 48·7. The fallacies involved in the acceptance of the mean age at death as a sanitary test will be stated at page 245.

Effect of Marital Condition.—Dr. Bertillon's tables, compiled from the returns of France from 1856–65, show that the death-rates of married adults are considerably lower than those of the unmarried, the death-rates for widows and widowers being the highest of all.

Death-Rate per 1,000 *Living of Married and Unmarried.*

Ages.	Males.			Females.		
	Single.	Married.	Widowers.	Single.	Married.	Widows.
20–25	12·88	8·92	49·60	8·32	9·92	12·31
25–30	10·17	6·24	21·84	9·02	8·98	23·62
30–35	11·51	6·82	19·17	9·87	9·36	16·90
35–40	13·15	7·52	17·50	10·87	9·29	15·03
40–45	16·62	9·55	18·89	13·28	10·14	12·73
45–50	19·60	11·47	22·20	15·71	19·69	13·30
50–55	25·80	15·61	26·80	20·97	14·11	15·20
55–60	32·10	21·50	34·17	26·90	19·29	24·47
60–65	45·92	32·60	47·50	40·52	30·75	37·07
65–70	58·50	44·80	62·97	58·30	45·30	53·50

Married life exposes women to the dangers of child-birth; but, spite of this fact, married women have a much lower mortality than spinsters, and still lower than widows. Although it is probable that married life is more conducive to longevity than single life, the proportionate salubrity of the two is not expressed by the proportion between the corresponding rates, in the above table. Although the influence of class is almost eliminated by the national character of the figures quoted, it may fairly be argued that, by a process of selection, it is the healthy men and women who chiefly marry, while the originally sickly are more likely to be found classed among the single.

The high rate for widowers aged 20-25, in comparison with bachelors and married men of the same age, may be largely due to accidental causes of difference. It should be remembered that the number of widowers aged 20-25 is comparatively small, and it is a sound rule in statistics that the smaller the number of individual facts on which a given rate per centum or per mille is founded, the less trustworthy is the result.

Effect of Sanitation.—The effect of density of population on mortality will be discussed in the next chapter. In view of the fact that such increased density tends to produce increased mortality, which we may assume for the present, and remembering that the population of England and Wales is every year becoming urban in a greater proportion, even a stationary rate of mortality cannot be regarded in any other light than as a cause of congratulation and not of reproach to sanitarians. Dr. Farr pointed this out in his 34th Report (1871). "In the last twenty years the towns of England have increased from 580 to 938, their population from 9 to 14 millions, and the health of the whole population has remained stationary." The same tendency to increased aggregation in cities is seen in France, where, in 1846, the urban population formed 24·4 per cent. of the entire population; in 1856, 27·3 per cent.; in 1866, 30·4 per cent.; and in 1872, 31·0 per cent.

The following table from the preliminary report of the 1881 census, shows the relative numbers of the country and town populations.

	Area in Acres.	Years.	Population Enumerated.	Increase in preceding Decennium.	Increase per cent. in preceding Decennium.
ENGLAND AND WALES . . .	37,319,321	1851	17 927,609	—	—
		1861	20 066,224	2,138,615	11·93
		1871	22,712,266	2,646,042	13·19
		1881	25,968,286	3,256,020	14·34
Town Population; i.e., inhabitants of the districts and sub-districts which include the chief towns . .	3,184,419	1851	9,155,964	—	—
		1861	10,933,234	1,777,270	19·41
		1871	12,910,647	1,977,413	18·09
		1881	15,444,808	2,534,161	19·63
Country Population; i.e., inhabitants of the remainder of England and Wales, which comprises the smaller towns and the country parishes . . .	34,134,302	1851	8,771,645	—	—
		1861	9,132,990	361,345	4·12
		1871	9,801,619	668,629	7·32
		1881	10,523,478	721,859	7·36

The following table shows in a succinct form the percentage of urban and rural populations at three decennial periods.

	Percentage of Population of England and Wales.		
	1861	1871	1881
Urban Population . . .	62·3	64·8	66·6
Rural Population	37·7	35·2	33·4

Now, although this steadily increasing amount of urban population would, according to natural laws, imply an increased mortality, up to 1871 the health of the whole country remained stationary. Since that time there has been a remarkable reduction in the death-rate, concerning which we cannot do better than quote the Registrar-General's report for 1881 (page xv. *et seq.*). "There is nothing in the series of annual reports issued by this office that comes out more distinctly and unmistakably than the wonderful effect which the sanitary operations of the last decade have had in saving life. The Public Health Act came into operation in 1872. The average annual death-rate for the immediately preceding ten years (1862–71) had been 22·6, and there were no indications whatsoever of any tendency of the rate to fall lower. Indeed in 1871, the final year of this period, the rate was exactly the average, viz., 22·6. The Act came into force, and at once the rate began to fall, and continued to fall year by year with almost unbroken regularity, until in 1881 it was no more than 18·9. Once only in the ten years that had elapsed since the Act came into operation was the rate as high as the average of the previous decade. That was in 1875, when the rate was 22·7. In that year a second Public Health Act, of more stringent character, came into operation; and from that date down to 1881 the death-rate did not once reach 22·0, and averaged no more than 20·5.

"Had the fall in the death-rate been limited to a single year, or to two years, or even to three, it might have been argued by sceptical persons that the improvement was due to a succession of seasons favourable to health, or to other causes unconnected with sanitary administration, and that the setting in of the fall coincidently with the coming into operation of public health measures was no more than casual; but in face of a fall, lasting for ten years in succession and increasing each year in amount, no one can seriously maintain such a position. There can be no real doubt that the saving effected in life was the direct product of the money and labour expended in sanitary improvements. Doubtless the money thus expended was enormous in amount; and it will be well, therefore, to consider what return it has brought in. If, then, the death-rate in 1881 had been only equal to the average death-rate in the decade preceding the Public Health Act of 1872, there would have died in the course of that one year 96,917 persons who, as it was, survived. From this total, however, a deduction must be made of some 5,000 for the following reason:—The birth-rate in 1881 and in each of the two immediately preceding years was considerably below the average annual birth-rate in 1862–71. Consequently there was a smaller than average proportion of children in the first three years of life in the population of 1881. But the death-rate at this early period of life is always very high. Had the birth-rate in 1879, 1880, 1881 been equal to the average birth-rate in 1862–71, there would have been so many more young children living in 1881 as to have increased the deaths in that year by a number close upon 5,000. Instead, therefore, of 96,917 lives saved, we have only about 92,000.

"Now we shall probably be well within the mark if we assume that for every fatal case of illness there are from four to five more cases which end in recovery. This is about the proportion in enteric fever, which is a more fatal disease than the average of diseases. The result, therefore, on this assumption, would be that, speaking in round numbers, there were 500,000 fewer cases of illness, and 92,000 fewer deaths in England and Wales in 1881 than would have been the case had the population been living under the conditions that existed in 1862–71. It may perhaps, be objected, and not unreasonably, that the year 1881, with its extraordinarily low death-rate, was so exceptional that it can hardly be taken as a fair sample by which to measure the annual return in life and health from the moneys spent in sanitary improvements. Let us then take the entire period of ten years that elapsed between the first Public Health Act and the close of 1881. Had the death-rate remained during that period at its mean level in the preceding decade, the total deaths from 1872 to 1881 inclusively would have been 5,548,116; whereas they were actually no more than 5,155,367. Thus no less than 392,749 persons who, under the old *régime*, would have died were, as a matter of fact, still living at the close of 1881. (The mean birth-rates in the two decades 1862–71 and 1872–81 were almost exactly the same, so that no correction need be made in this case). Add to these saved lives the avoidance of at least four times as many attacks of non-fatal illness, and we have the total profits as yet received from our sanitary expenditure. Moreover, it is important to note that these profits were not equally spread over the ten years, but that there was a manifest tendency to progressive increase throughout the period. This is what might be anticipated; for the full effect of sanitary improvements requires time for development." We may add that if the death-rates between 1881 and 1888 are included, the improvement realized becomes even more striking. Thus—

	Period of Years.	Mean Annual Death-Rate per 1,000 Living.
	Ten Years, 1862–71	22·6
Public Health Act, 1872—	Four Years, 1872–75	21·8
Public Health Act, 1875—	Five Years, 1876–80	20·79
	Five Years, 1881–85	19·30
	1886	19·28
	1887	18·79
	1888	17·83

In the decennium 1871-80, the mean annual death-rate varied from 14·13 to 33·57 per 1,000 in different districts. During this period England and Wales were divided, for registration purposes, into 647 districts, in 8 of which the mean annual death-rate was under 15 per 1,000; in 31, under 16 per 1,000; and in 62, did not exceed 17 per 1,000. These 101 districts constitute what are called the *Selected Healthy Districts,* and form a convenient standard of comparison. In 326 districts the death-rate was between 17 and 20; in 195, between 20 and 25; in 23, between 25 and 30 per 1,000; and in the remaining two exceeded the last figure. Dr. Ogle points out that it would not be fair to assume that the differences between these different districts are due to the varying efficiency with which the Public Health Act is carried out; and that apart from the slight differences due to geological and climatic influences, these districts should have an equal mortality. While it is true that there is a great and general decline in mortality since active efforts have been made at sanitation, and that this decline is greatest in the districts where sanitary administration has been most active (greater in the urban than in the rural districts), other factors of excessive mortality, over which sanitary authorities have little or no control, must be remembered—as poverty, crime, drunkenness, unhealthy occupations, and the degree of aggregation of the population.

The report made by Dr. Buchanan to the Privy Council in 1867 on twenty-five towns, having an aggregate population of 606,186 inhabitants, shows very strikingly the influence of definite sanitary works on the mortality from typhoid fever and from phthisis. The sanitary improvements in these towns included drainage of houses and of the surface and subsoil; improved water supply; measures for removing decomposing organic matters, for improved paving and scavenging and public cleanliness, and for the amendment of lodging-houses and the repression of overcrowding. The following table gives a few illustrations of the effect of such sanitary works from Dr. Buchanan's more extensive table.

Effect of Sanitary Works on the General Death-Rate and on the Mortality from Typhoid Fever and Phthisis.

Towns.	Death-Rate before Construction of Works.	Death-Rate after Construction of Works.	Reduction of Typhoid per Cent.	Reduction of Phthisis per Cent.
Banbury . .	23·4	20·5	48	41
Cardiff . .	33·2	22·6	40	17
Croydon . .	23·7	18·6	63	17
Dover . . .	22·6	20·9	36	20
Ely	23·9	20·5	56	47
Leicester . .	26·4	25·2	48	32
Macclesfield .	29·8	23·7	48	31
Merthyr . .	33·2	26·2	60	11
Newport . .	31·8	21·6	36	32
Rugby . .	19·1	18·6	10	43
Salisbury . .	27·5	21·9	75	49
Warwick . .	22·7	21·0	52	19

In these twelve towns the average death-rate was lowered

from 25·6 to 21·7 per 1,000; the mortality from typhoid fever was reduced 10–75 per cent., and from phthisis 11–49 per cent.

The facts stated in the preceding table may be compared with Dr. Kelly's figures (page 120). There can be no question as to the great diminution of phthisis in this country, and that this is due to sanitary improvements. It is worthy of note that Mr. (now Sir John) Simon, commenting on Dr. Buchanan's results in his report for 1867 to the Privy Council, while thinking that there is no possibility of questioning the conclusion that dampness of soil is an important cause of phthisis to the population living on the soil, is careful to state that this conclusion does not purport to be more than a contribution to the etiology of phthisis. He points out that the disease has an industrial aspect, that its hereditary relations are important, and that the infective nature of the morbid process accompanying it requires elucidation.

Mortality at School Ages.—The influence of the present educational system on the health of children in this country is so important a question that no apology is necessary for quoting the following statement from the Registrar-General's Annual Report for 1882.

" We have no means of giving the death-rates of children of the precise ages 3–13, as requested, for this age-period is not one that is used by us in abstracting deaths. We can, however, give the death-rate of children of from 5 to 15 years of age, and this age-period will probably be a better one than 3–13 to test the possible effect of school-work on children's mortality; for, though the children of three and four years of age are omitted, school can scarcely be supposed to affect them in the way of injury from overwork; and, though boys and girls of 14 and 15 are included, it must be remembered that any injurious effects of overwork at school that may exist will be carried on after the actual school attendance is finished. The effect, if there be any, of overwork would be in the latter years of school attendance; viz., the 12th and 13th years, and the injury would cause increased mortality, not only in those years, but at least for some few years afterwards. The age-period, then, which we take is the decade from 5 to 15 years of age, and the periods we take for comparison are the decennia 1861–70 and 1871–80.

"The death-rate of children (5–15) in 1861–70 was 6·3 per 1,000. It fell in 1871–80 to 5·1 per 1,000; a decline of 19·05 per cent. The main part in this fall was due to diminished mortality from the chief zymotic diseases; namely, small-pox, measles, scarlatina, whooping-cough, diphtheria, fever, and diarrhœa. These diseases caused a mortality of 2·9 per 1,000 in the first decennial period, but only of 2·1 per 1,000 in the second.

"But after excluding these diseases from the account as irrelative to the question at issue, there was still a considerable decline in mortality. In the first period (1861–70) the death-rate from all causes other than zymotic was 3·4 per 1,000; in the second it was only 3·0.

"But inasmuch as school work, if it be injurious to health, would probably be so by affecting the brain and, generally, the nervous system, it would be well to split up these death-rates from causes other than zymotic, into death-rates from diseases of the nervous system and death-rates from other causes. When this is done, we find that the entire fall was due to diminished mortality from other causes. The rate from these fell from 2·9 to 2·5 per 1,000, whereas the death-rate from nervous affections remained unaffected. Indeed, if a second place of decimals were taken, it would appear that nervous diseases had slightly, very slightly, increased.

"It would appear, therefore, that, while the mortality of children from all causes and from zymotic causes has considerably diminished, their mortality from diseases of the nervous system has exceptionally remained stationary. The general improvement has not affected this class of diseases.

Annual Death-Rate per 1,000 *living of Children aged* 5–15 *in England and Wales in the two decades* 1861–70 *and* 1871–80.

Years.	All Causes.	Principal Zymotic Diseases.	Diseases of Nervous System.	Other Causes.
1861–70	6·3	2·9	0·5	2·9
1871–80	5·1	2·1	0·5	2·5

"To the above answer to the question addressed to this office may now be added the supplementary fact that the figures for 1881 and 1882 also showed a further and considerable decline in the deaths of children of the ages in question from all causes together, and from the chief zymotic diseases, while their death-rate from nervous diseases remained in each of the two years at exactly the same point as in the two preceding decades."

"It may also be well to note that tubercular meningitis or acute hydrocephalus is not included in the foregoing table among diseases of the nervous system; and that the mortality ascribed to this cause was somewhat higher in 1881 and 1882 than in 1861–70. Both in 1881 and 1882 the death-rate among children of school age from this cause was 0·22 per 1,000, whereas in 1861–70 it averaged 0·20."

These statistics undoubtedly appear to give countenance to the view that the strain of education produces in a certain proportion of children injurious effects on the nervous system. It would, however, be unsafe to draw certain conclusions from these figures. The medical certificates of death relating to children are often ambiguous in statement, and the absence of any decrease in diseases of the nervous system may be due to accidental causes of variation and not to the influence of school-life. The whole question of "overpressure" is discussed in my manual of *School Hygiene.*

CHAPTER IX.

DENSITY OF POPULATION AND MORTALITY.

Estimation of Degree of Aggregation.—Relation between Density and Mortality.—Urban and Rural Population.—Urban and Rural Mortality. —Apparent and Real Differences.—Effect of Density on Mortality of Young.—Range of Action of Density on Mortality.—Effect of Higher Degrees of Density on Mortality.—Size of House and Mortality.—Artisans' Block Buildings.—Back to Back Houses.—Causes of High Mortality from Increased Density.—Impure Air.—Infectious Diseases. —Phthisis.—Poverty and Drunkenness.

DR. FARR first called attention to the influence exerted by density of population on mortality in the fifth Report of the Registrar-General (1843), and since that time the relationship between density and mortality has been further elucidated.

Method of Estimating Degree of Aggregation of Population. —Two methods are commonly adopted. (1) The number of persons living to each square mile of area is stated. (2) The average number of acres occupied by each person in the population is stated.

The following table gives an example of both these methods:—

England and Wales—Density and Mortality.

	1841-50	1851-60.	1861-70.	1871-80.
Death-Rate per 1,000	22	22	22	21·3
Persons to a Square Mile	—	325	365	415
Acres to a Person (Mean Density) .	2·21	1·96	1·74	1·53

If Area$=$A, and population$=$P,

Then $\frac{P}{A}$=D=mean population on each unit of area,

While $\frac{A}{P}$=the mean area to each person.

The unit of space in the first method is taken to be a mile; in the second (so that whole numbers may be secured), an acre.

Relation between Density and Mortality.—Dr. Farr found that the mortality increases with the density of the population, but not in direct proportion to their densities, but as their 6th root.

Thus if d and d'=density of population in two places,
and m and m'=mortality " " "

$$\text{then } \frac{m'}{m} = \sqrt[6]{\frac{d'}{d}}$$

$$\text{and } m' : m :: \sqrt[6]{d'} : \sqrt[6]{d}$$

In his report for 1843, Dr. Farr gives as examples seven groups of districts the death-rate of which, calculated from their densities, approximated very closely to the observed death-rates. Thus—

Death-Rates—

Calculated:	18·90—19·16—20·87—25·02—28·08—37·70—38·74.
Observed:	16·75—19·16—21·88—24·90—28·08—32·49—38·62.

The formula was subsequently altered by Dr. Farr (Supplement to 35th Annual Report, page clviii.), 0·11998 being substituted for $\frac{1}{6}$ in the above formula; or, more exactly—

$$m' = m\left(\frac{d'}{d}\right)^{0·11998}$$

Thus in 1861–70, in the 345 districts, which had a mortality of 19·2, the density was 186 persons to a square mile; in the 9 districts with a density of 4,499, what was the mortality? It was happily not expressed by the proportion of the two densities; *i.e.*, 186 : 4,499 :: 19·2 : x; but by this proportion nearly—

$$(186)^{0·12} : (4{,}499)^{0·12} :: 19·2 : x = 28·1.$$

This formula only gives slightly different results from the preceding one. So closely was the ratio found to be followed in places whose sewage and water supply and other sanitary conditions were fairly the same, and which apparently differed only in density of population, that Dr. Farr went so far as to propose that in any sanitary inquiry the influence of density should first be discovered by means of the above formula, and that the effect of other influences above or below this should then be investigated. As he remarks, "the formula thus eliminates the element of density from the analysis of the causes of insalubrity."

Urban and Rural Population.—From what has been already said, it would appear that "urbanization" tends greatly to neutralize the effects of sanitation. We have seen (page 125), that the percentage of urban population is steadily on the increase, while the rural population shows a corresponding decrease. It should be noted that the *urban population* consists of the inhabitants of the chief towns and their immediate vicinities, while the *rural population* includes the inhabitants of the smaller towns, as well as the strictly country parishes. Using the words in this sense, the urban stood to the remaining or rural population in 1881 in the proportion of 147 to 100; the proportion in 1871 having been 132 to 100. The rural population thus determined includes the inhabitants of a very large number of places, which although not large enough to rank as "chief towns," are yet of such a size that their inhabitants can scarcely be said to live under rural conditions. The division of the country into **sanitary areas** affords the best basis for calculating what would be the urban population if made to include these. At the time of the census of 1881 there were 967 urban sanitary districts, besides the 39 districts within the jurisdiction of the Metropolitan Board of Works; the aggregate population of these 1,006 districts being 17,648,354, while that of the remaining rural sanitary districts amounted to 8,319,932; the proportion between the two being, therefore, as 212 to 100. Among these urban sanitary districts, however, some are of such small dimensions that they should be excluded from the list. If all districts with a smaller population than 3,000 are excluded, 771 urban sanitary districts are left (reckoning London as one), the constitution of which is shown in the following table:—

Urban Sanitary Districts in 1881 with Population of	Number of Districts.	Aggregate Population, 1881.	Percentage of Population of England & Wales, 1881.
100,000 and upwards	20 (including London)	7,696,132	29·7
50 000–100,000	28	1,850,088	7·1
20,000–50,000	96	2,883,702	11·1
10,000–20,000	160	2,214,366	8·5
3,000–10,000	467	2,640,738	10·2
Total Urban Population	771	17,285,026	66·6
Total Rural Population	—	8,683,260	33·4
Population of England and Wales .	—	25,968,286	100·0

The following figures represent approximately the respective growths of the present urban and rural populations, as constituted in the preceding table.

	Percentage of Population of England and Wales.		
	1861.	1871.	1881.
Urban Population . . .	62·3	64·8	66·6
Rural Population . . .	37·7	35·2	33·4

Urban and Rural Mortality.—The table given on page 116 gives the death-rate in town and country districts for each quarter of several years. The urban is invariably higher than the rural mortality, the difference being usually least in the second quarter of the year and greatest in the third and fourth quarters. In the ten years 1874–83, if the mean rural mortality in each quarter be represented as 100, the urban mortality was, in the four successive quarters, beginning with the first, 116, 112, 128 and 127. In the table referred to, and in the following table, the rural and urban districts are constituted as defined in the table at page 116.

Death-Rates in Town and Country Districts of England, 1851-86.

Year.	Persons to a Square Mile in England and Wales.	Annual Deaths to 1,000 Persons Living in			Deaths in Town Districts to 100 Deaths in Country Districts, in Equal Numbers Living.
		England and Wales.	Town Districts.	Country Districts.	
1851–60 . .	325	22·2	24·7	19·9	124
1861–70 . .	365	22·5	24·8	19·7	126
1871–80 . .	415	21·4	23·1	19·0	122
1881 . . .	447	18·9	20·1	16·9	119
1882 . . .	454	19·6	20·9	17·3	121
1883 . . .	460	19·5	20·5	17·9	115
1884 . . .	466	19·5	20·6	17·7	117
1885 . . .	473	19·0	19·7	17·8	111
1886 . . .	479	19·3	20·0	18·0	111

In 1886, while the urban death-rate was 20·0, the rural death-rate was only 18·0 per 1,000 living. The difference between the two is, however, as shown by the last column of the preceding table, steadily decreasing; for while the urban rate before the present decennium had been 22 to 26 per cent. above the rural rate, the excess fell to 11 per cent. in 1886, although in this year summer diarrhœa, a specially urban disease, was more than usually prevalent.

The *true difference* between urban and rural mortality is greater than is shown in the preceding tables, if due allowance be made for age and sex distribution. There is in towns (*a*) a much larger proportion of females, (*b*) a larger proportion of adults of both sexes in the prime of life, and (*c*) a much smaller proportion of very aged persons, who commonly retire to the country. There is the slightly counterbalancing influence of a large number of infants in towns; but these, as shown before (page 70), are followed by an increase of young adults, and, therefore, *apart from any excess of infantile mortality*, ought not to raise the general rate of mortality. The extent of the correction required on this account may be gathered from an example. In 1884 the urban death-rate was 20·6; the rural death-rate 17·7. Owing however to the great differences of age and sex-distribution of the respective populations, the urban death-rate ought, with equal healthiness, to have been nearly 11 per cent. lower than the rural death-rate, instead of being, as it was, 20·1 per cent. above it.

Similarly, in the decennium 1871–80, taking as a standard the mean death-rates at each age-period in England and Wales for the decennium, the general death-rate in urban districts should have been 20·4 (instead of 23·1), and in rural districts should have been 22·83 per 1,000 (instead of 19·0), that of England and Wales being 21·7. That is, assuming that the urban and rural populations were equally healthy, the death-rate of the former should have been 4·09 per cent. below, and that of the latter 7·33 per cent. above, the mortality of England and Wales.

Effect of Density on Mortality of Young.—The ill effects of increased aggregation of population are much greater in the earlier years of life. This is clearly shown by the following figures (Supplement to 35th Report, p. clx.).

Persons to a Square Mile	166	186	379	1,718	4,499	12,357	65,823
Death-Rate at all Ages .	16·94	19·18	21·90	24·81	28·02	32·92	38·67
Death-Rate under Five .	37·80	47·53	63·06	82·10	94·04	111·90	139·52

The figures in the last vertical column refer to the Liverpool district. Comparing these figures with those for 64 healthy selected districts (with a mortality of 15–17 per 1,000 living, and comprising a population of about one million people), we find that while the death-rate for all ages is increased 128·3 per cent., the death-rate under five is increased 269·1 per cent.; *i.e.*, to every 100 deaths at all ages, and to every 100 deaths under five in healthy districts, there were during 1861–70 in Liverpool 228 deaths at all ages and 369 deaths under five respectively.

Range of Action of Density on Mortality.—In individual cases there is occasional difficulty in determining whether an open area within a sanitary district ought to form part of its true area. The population may be lodged on only a portion of the area of a district, the remaining area being occupied by a lake, common, park, etc. The usual plan adopted is to include these (thus diminishing the apparent density of population) if they are within the borders of the sanitary district.

The following table, from Dr. Ogle's supplement to the 45th Annual Report of the Registrar-General, illustrates the connection between aggregation of population and death-rate:—

Groups of Districts arranged according to Density and Death-Rates, 1871–80.

Annual Death-Rate per 1000.	Number of Districts.	Ten years, 1871-80. Mean Population.	Deaths.	Mean Annual death-rate per 1000.	Mean Density (Acres to a Person).	Persons to a Square Mile.
Cols	1.	2.	3.	4.	5.	6.
14 and under 15	8	171,244	24,804	14·48	2·53	253
15 ,, ,, 16	31	503,594	78,570	15·60	3·20	200
16 ,, ,, 17	62	1,379,250	229,301	16·63	2·48	258
17 ,, ,, 18	102	2,166,690	380,980	17·58	3·04	211
18 ,, ,, 19	129	2,787,836	516,671	18·53	3·30	194
19 ,, ,, 20	95	2,308,721	449,736	19·48	2·94	217
20 ,, ,, 21	50	2,450,483	503,702	20·56	1·40	458
21 ,, ,, 22	46	2,551,807	549,573	21·54	0·95	677
22 ,, ,, 23	42	2,692,101	607,008	22·55	0·49	1,301
23 ,, ,, 24	30	2,666,484	627,660	23·54	0·35	1,819
24 ,, ,, 25	27	2,088,340	509,661	24·41	0·30	2,166
25 ,, ,, 26	14	1,375,652	351,318	25·54	0·23	2,819
26 ,, ,, 27	5	350,681	92,092	26·26	0·22	2,944
27 ,, ,, 34	6	850,906	257,247	30·23	0·10	6,141

In this table the districts have been classified in the order of their recorded death-rates. If the death-rates were determined simply by degree of density of population, Dr. Ogle points out that the series of figures in col. 6 would of course increase regularly from the top downwards, as do the rates in col. 4; and this is actually the case for the latter and much greater part of the column, but there is considerable irregularity in the first few terms of the series. Apparently only after the density has reached a certain degree of intensity does it begin to exert an appreciable effect. "This might have been anticipated. For though in crowded communities it may be a matter of vital importance whether there are 500, or 1,000, or 2,000, or more persons living on a square mile, yet it can scarcely make any difference, so far as health goes, whether in rural districts there be two acres or three acres on an average to each inhabitant. The differences in the death-rates in these sparse populations are determined by other conditions than aggregation."

Effects of Higher Degrees of Density on Mortality.—No better illustration of the evils connected with overcrowding can be given than that furnished by Dr. J. B. Russell in his address to the Glasgow Philosophical Society (November, 1888). He brings out very strikingly the connection between size of the average house and the general death-rate. Aberdeen, which has 13·6 per cent. of its population living in one room, has the lowest death-rate of eight great Scotch towns, the death-rate rising *pari passu* with the diminution in size of the average house, until we come to Glasgow with 24·7 per cent. of its population living in one room, and the highest death-rate. In comparing the twenty-four districts into which Glasgow is divided, the same general relation is demonstrated. The population of Glasgow in 1885 was 543,295, the number of deaths 13,439. The distribution of population and deaths in the inhabited houses according to their size was as follows:—

Size of House.	Population.	Deaths.	Percentage of Population.	Percentage of Deaths.
One Room	134,728	3,636	24·7	27·0
Two Rooms	243,691	6,325	44·7	47·0
Three "	86,956	1,747	16·0	13·0
Four "	32,742	581	6·1	4·3
Five Rooms and upwards	38,647	434	7·1	3·3
Institutions	6,531	427	1·4	3·2
Untraced	—	289	—	2·2
Whole city	543,295	13,439	100·0	100·0

It will be seen that in both one and two-room houses the deaths were 2·3 per cent. above the due proportion, while in the houses above this size they were all below the due proportion in varying degree. The difference between the distribution of population and deaths may be seen at a glance from Dr. Russell's diagram.

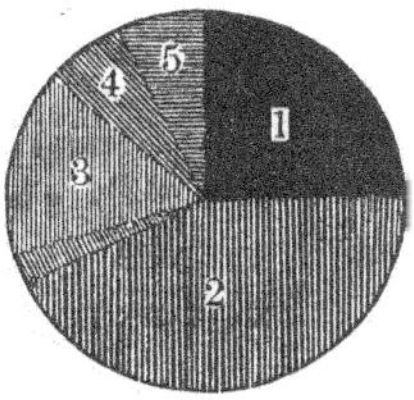

Population.

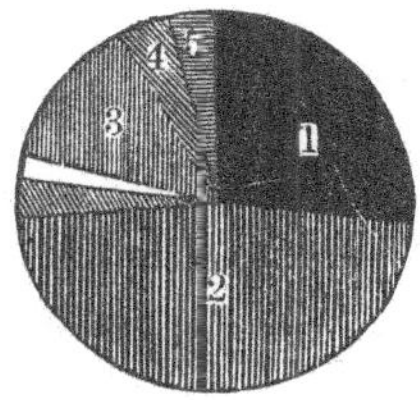

Deaths.

The one and two-room houses mentioned above are commonly "made-down houses," *i.e.*, parts of houses of larger size, which are now let separately. In some cases single rooms are divided by wood partitions, and let to two separate families.

If the *death-rates* in these various classes of the population be compared—the deaths in institutions and the unallocated deaths being placed, as in the diagram, along with the deaths contributed by one and two-room houses—it will be found that among those living in one and two-room houses, the death-rate is 27·74 per 1000; among those living in houses of three and four rooms, 19·45; and among those living in houses of five rooms and upwards, only 11·23.

Next as to the *incidence of certain classes of disease* upon these sections of the population, Dr. Russell selected zymotic diseases; diseases of the lungs, including consumption; diseases special to children under five years of age (as convulsions and other diseases of the nervous system, atrophy or wasting, and premature birth); deaths of children from accident and syphilitic disease, "a small class, but one pregnant with meaning." In the following table the rates per 100,000 inhabitants from each of these are shown:—

	One and Two-Room Houses.	Three and Four-Room Houses.	Five Rooms and upwards.
Zymotic Diseases	478	246	114
Acute Diseases of the Lungs (including Consumption) . . .	985	689	328
Nervous Diseases and Diseases of Nutrition in children	480	235	91
Accidents and Syphilis in children	32	11	—
Miscellaneous Unclassified Diseases	799	764	590
All Causes	2,774	1,945	1,123

The same results are exhibited in the following diagram, in which the three columns being drawn on the same scale, the comparative general death-rate in the three grades of houses, as well as the comparative prevalence of these classes of disease can be seen by the height of the columns and their different positions.

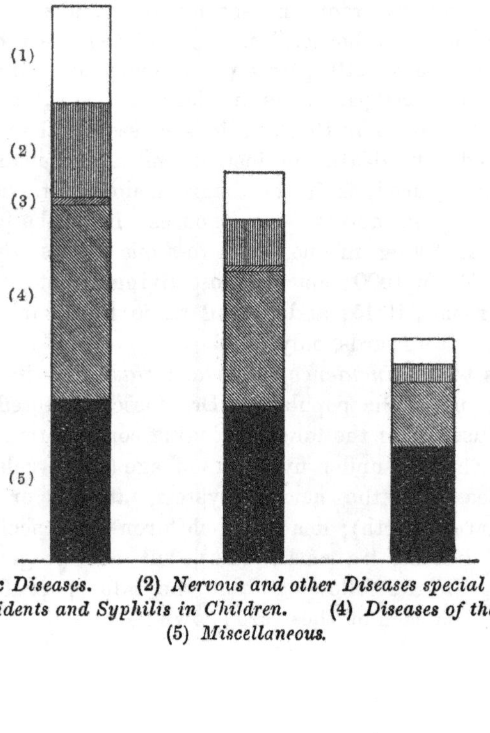

(1) *Zymotic Diseases.* (2) *Nervous and other Diseases special to Children.* (3) *Accidents and Syphilis in Children.* (4) *Diseases of the Lungs.* (5) *Miscellaneous.*

Glasgow forms an instance of a dense population under insanitary conditions. It would be a mistake, however, to suppose that the ratio of density to mortality demonstrated by Dr. Farr is an inexorable law incapable of mitigation. The fact that the urban death-rate, is generally decreasing in spite of increasing density, and is decreasing at a more rapid rate than the rural death-rate, is a disproof of this. In the following table there is no constant relationship between the density of population and the height of the death-rate in the twenty-eight great towns of England and Wales:—

CITIES AND BOROUGHS.	BIRTHS in 52 Weeks ending 2nd Jan., 1887.	Total Deaths. 52 or 53 Weeks ending				POPULATION, Estimated to the middle of 1887.	Persons to an Acre.
		3rd Jan., 1885.	2nd Jan., 1886.	1st Jan., 1887.	31st Dec., 1887.		
Cols.	1.	2.	3.	4.	5.	6.	7.
28 Towns . . .	32·2	21·6	20·6	20·9	20·8	9,244,099	36·9
London	31·7	20·4	19·8	19·9	19·6	4,215,192	56·0
Brighton . . .	25·8	18·0	17·1	17·1	16·9	118,186	47·0
Portsmouth . .	36·8	19·4	19·7	23·8	19·5	137,917	31·9
Norwich . . .	33·9	21·2	20·3	23·3	20·4	92,848	12·4
Plymouth . . .	31·5	21·0	22·3	23·5	22·7	77,127	52·5
Bristol	29·7	18·4	19·7	19·3	20·4	223,695	48·3
Wolverhampton .	33·2	23·4	20·2	22·2	21·7	80,847	23·8
Birmingham . .	31·8	21·4	19·3	19·9	19·7	441,095	52·5
Leicester . . .	32·8	22·1	19·8	20·3	19·5	143,153	44·7
Nottingham . .	33·3	22·9	19·9	20·4	18·7	224,230	22·5
Derby	30·0	18·4	18·1	18·2	17·1	94,006	27·2
Birkenhead . .	32·5	19·6	19·5	19·1	21·0	97,703	25·4
Liverpool . . .	31·2	25·2	23·8	23·8	23·7	592,991	113·8
Bolton	32·5	24·1	20·8	23·1	21·3	112,354	46·7
Manchester . .	35·9	26·4	26·5	26·3	28·7	377,529	87·9
Salford	31·9	22·3	21·1	22·1	22·2	218,658	42·3
Oldham	31·3	24·5	22·0	22·8	23·8	134,158	28·4
Blackburn . . .	35·8	24·1	21·8	25·5	25·5	116,844	16·8
Preston	38·5	27·3	27·1	28·9	27·9	102,283	27·5
Huddersfield . .	27·7	19·6	20·1	19·6	23·0	90,034	8·6
Halifax	28·4	23·4	19·7	22·8	21·0	79,207	21·0
Bradford . . .	27·7	20·1	17·7	19·2	19·9	224,507	20·8
Leeds	33·3	24·2	19·9	21·9	21·1	345,080	16·0
Sheffield . . .	32·9	22·4	20·7	19·8	21·6	316,288	16·1
Hull	32·8	21·1	17·2	18·8	19·2	196,855	24·9
Sunderland . .	34·6	23·1	23·8	19·5	19·7	129,684	42·8
Newcastle . . .	39·1	23·1	26·1	22·2	25·3	157,048	29·2
Cardiff	41·1	24·4	25·7	22·6	21·9	104,580	14·2

The **Peabody and Artisans' Block Buildings** in London may be taken as an instance of a large number of tenements massed on a very small area, and yet arranged so that each shall receive sufficient air, and fulfil all other sanitary requirements. In 1884 there were 10,144 living rooms provided in the Peabody Buildings, occupied by 18,453 persons. The birth-rate was 44·6 per 1,000, or 10·9 higher than the rate for all London. This is good evidence that the population of the Peabody Buildings was of an age-distribution favourable to a low death-rate. The recorded death-rate corrected for hospitals was 19·1 per 1,000, or 1·2 below the general death-rate of London. The infantile mortality was 138·7 per 1,000 births, 13·7 below the average for London. It cannot be denied, however, that the population in these buildings is to some extent a selected one, and that the weakly and old are drafted from them. At the present time (1888) over 100,000 people are housed in Artisans' Block Buildings, and it may be hoped that ere long trustworthy vital statistics concerning them, making due allowance for favourable age-constitution of their population, will be forthcoming.

Back-to-Back Houses illustrate very clearly the effect of close aggregation of population, involving as it does in this case deficient light and ventilation, and imperfect sanitary arrangements. This practice of building houses back to back, and therefore without provision for through ventilation, is common in many Yorkshire and Lancashire towns. The most trustworthy statistics bearing on the subject are those furnished by Mr. Gordon Smith and Dr. Barry in their report on **Back-to-Back** Houses. Of course other factors may have influenced the results shown in the following table besides the presence or absence of through ventilation, as the arrangement of the streets, the sanitary surroundings of the houses, social status of the inhabitants, etc.

The Greengates and Regent Road registration sub-districts of Salford were each divided into three groups, as shown in the following table, which will enable the relative mortality of each from various special causes to be seen at a glance :—

		Population.	Death-rate per 1,000 living from				
			All Causes.	Pulmonary Diseases, excluding Phthisis.	Phthisis.	Seven Chief Zymotic Diseases.	Diarrhœa.
Greengates Sub-District	Group I.—No back-to-back houses	8,713	27·5	6·6	2·8	4·5	1·42
	Group II.—Average proportion of 23 per cent. of back-to-back houses	11,749	29·2	7·8	3·3	4·8	1·55
	Group III.—Average proportion of 56 per cent. of back-to-back houses	11,405	30·5	7·9	3·6	6·2	2·12
Regent Road Sub-District	Group I.—No back-to-back houses	54,264	26·1	5·7	2·7	4·9	1·54
	Group II.—Average proportion of 18 per cent. of back-to-back houses	8,773	29·1	7·5	2·7	4·9	1·85
	Group III.—Average proportion of 50 per cent. of back-to-back houses	4,380	37·3	8·6	4·5	7·6	2·83

It will be seen that the mortality from all causes, from pulmonary diseases, from phthisis, and from the seven chief zymotic diseases taken together, as well as from diarrhœa alone, increase *pari passu* with the proportion of back-to-back houses.

Causes of High Mortality with Increased Density.—The higher death-rates, which go hand in hand with increased density of population, are not the direct results of the latter. The crowding of persons together doubtless leads to the risks of fouling of air and water and soil, and to the increased propagation of infectious diseases, and thus directly affects the mortality. But these "direct consequences of close aggregation are probably as nothing in comparison with its indirect consequences or concomitants. The more crowded a community, the greater, speaking generally, is the amount of abject want, of filth, of crime, of drunkenness, and of other excesses, the more keen is the competition, and the more feverish and exhausting the conditions of life; moreover, and perhaps more than all, it is in these crowded communities that almost all the most dangerous and unhealthy industries are carried on. It is not so much the aggregation itself, as these other factors which are associated with aggregation, that produce the high mortality of our great towns or other thickly populated areas" (Ogle).

(1) Of the direct influences connected with close aggregation of population, *filth conditions* of air and water and soil are the most important. If the source of water supply is pure and the drainage is good, densely populated towns may be, and are, commonly better off in these matters than rural districts. But atmospheric impurities, especially in the form of decomposing organic matter, are doubtless more rife in town than in country; and Dr. Farr rightly lays special stress on these. Even in towns the amount of such impurities varies greatly in houses of different sizes, and such differences throw a flood of light on the facts already given regarding the higher mortality in one and two-room houses. The following table, given in a paper which appeared in the Philosophical Transactions for 1887, by Professor Carnelly and Drs. Haldane and Anderson, as the result of elaborate observations made at Dundee, shows very strikingly the differences in houses of varying size. Taking the average amount (in excess of outside air) of carbonic acid, organic matter, and micro-organisms, respectively, in the atmosphere of houses of four or more rooms as unity, then in one and two-room houses, the relative amount was as follows:—

	Houses of Four Rooms and upwards.	Two-room Houses.	One-room Houses.
Cubic Space per person . .	1	0·13	0·11
Carbonic Acid	1	1·5	2·0
Organic Matter	1	1·6	4·4
Micro-Organisms, total . .	1	5·1	6·7
Bacteria	1	3·1	6·9
Moulds	1	5·5	3·0

(2) The more rapid spread of *infectious diseases* is shown by the higher zymotic mortality in large towns, their more rapid

spread being partly due to the shorter distance the infection has to travel from individual to individual, and partly, also, to the fact that a fouled state of the atmosphere and soil facilitates the propagation of infection.

(3) Other diseases, as *phthisis*, are more common in urban than in rural districts. The close connection between phthisis and a foul atmosphere is well established. Dr. Anderson's researches in Dundee, and Dr. Russell's in Glasgow, both show that the mortality from phthisis in these towns is highest among the inmates of three-room houses; and the explanation suggested by the former is probably correct, that the high infantile mortality from other forms of tubercular disease returned as nervous diseases, atrophy, wasting, etc., prevents the growth of young adults (who are most prone to tubercle of the lungs) in the smaller houses.

(4) *Poverty* of the inhabitants of densely populated districts, implying as it does inadequate food and deficient clothing and shelter, has a great effect in swelling their mortality. Dr. Drysdale, in a paper read at the meeting of the British Medical Association in 1887, quotes as evidence of the importance of indigence as a cause of a high death-rate the lower mean age at death of the working classes (this is fallacious; see page 314); and the fact that in France 65 per 1,000 deaths among the rich are due to tubercular diseases, and 250 per 1,000 among the poor. In Dublin, Dr. Grimshaw states that in 1886 the death-rate per 1,000 living was 13·4 among the independent and professional classes, and 33·7 among the "service classes."

(5) *Other evil social conditions* commonly accompany poverty. Cities are commonly the hotbeds of vice and misery, of crime and drunkenness, as well as of filth and want. The Select Committee on Intemperance (4th Report, 1878) say: "On the whole, in the towns where the drunkenness is greatest, the population is most dense." The density of population and the drunkenness each of them probably stands in the place of both cause and effect.

Accidents are more common and more fatal in cities than in the country. The evil influences of *heredity* should also be mentioned, the organism tending to degenerate when placed, generation after generation, in an unwholesome environment.

(6) The influence of *occupation* and of homes involving exposure to poisonous effluvia and other poisonous agencies will be considered in the next chapter.

CHAPTER X.

EFFECT OF OCCUPATION ON MORTALITY.

Class and Occupation.—Difficulties of Classification.—Methods of Comparison between Occupations.—Fallacies of Mean Age at Death.—Dr. Ogle on Occupational Mortality.—Sources of Possible Error.—Mortality in Individual Occupations.—Comparative Mortality Figures.—Causes of Mortality in Different Occupations.—Influence of Foul Air and Dust.—Alcoholism and Lead-Poisoning.

CLASS and Occupation.—At the census of 1841 and more completely at the subsequent census enumerations, each individual was classified under his principal occupation on the census day, with distinction of age and sex. The distinction of age is important, as it enables us to compare the number living in each well-defined occupation with the number who are registered as dying at the corresponding ages, and thus to determine the influence of occupation on health and life; and also because it enables us to determine whether those engaged in any particular occupation are children, or young or old adults, which information has important social bearings. Twenty-four orders of occupation are described by the Registrar-General, which comprise 80 sub-orders or genera. The orders are grouped into six classes; viz., professional, domestic, commercial, agricultural, industrial, and non-productive.* The population may be divided roughly into two great groups,—those who work, and those who professedly have no definite occupation. After due allowance has been made for those who are infirm, or have retired in advanced age from their occupations, the number belonging to the second class in this country

* See Appendix I. (p. 315) for a tabular statement of the number following each of these groups of occupations.

is not great. Whatever classification of occupations is adopted, errors must occur, largely owing to ambiguity in the nomenclature of occupations. One great source of difficulty is the occurrence in the same individual of *double occupations.* The same person may be a farmer and a miller, or a plumber and gasfitter. In the 1851 census, the enumerators were instructed to this effect, that "a person following more than one distinct trade may insert his occupations in the order of their importance"; the first occupation being taken in the subsequent classification.

Another great source of difficulty is in *the separation of classes.* Condition of class may have as much to do with disease and mortality as occupation, but it is very difficult to separate, for instance, between masters and men in any given trade or manufacture. A watchmaker or tailor may be either a master or journeyman, the health conditions in the latter case being probably much more unfavourable than in the former; and similarly in other cases. Domestic servants, again, may be of all grades. Other instances will be given subsequently. Where possible, therefore, class, as well as occupation, should be distinctly stated in both the census and death-returns.

Two tests have been proposed as a criterion of class, or social status, in addition to that of occupation (1) the *rent of the dwelling* in which a family lives, which Dr. Rumsey regards as probably the nearest ascertainable test or index of prosperity. This, taken in conjunction with occupation, would decide and correct uncertain results, which now belong to the category of what have been called "conjectural statistics."

(2) *The number of rooms occupied* by each family. We have already (page 140) given an instance of investigation conducted on this basis, which Dr. Russell, of Glasgow, considers more certain and uniform in its results than one founded on rental; and in crowded neighbourhoods it furnishes interesting and useful statistics.

Methods of Comparison between Occupations.—(1) The mean ages at death of those engaged in different occupations are contrasted. This often, however, gives erroneous indications. The mean age at death is governed by the mean age of the living, and it is as much affected by the ages at which people enter and leave any given occupation, and by the increase or decrease of employment, as by its relative salubrity or insalubrity. In a large printing firm known to the writer, all the older *employés* have been discharged, and youths from fifteen to twenty-five years of age have taken their places at lower wages. Such a proceeding will obviously lower the mean age at death, but will by no means demonstrate that this particular printing establishment is carried on under less healthy conditions than formerly.

(2) The proportion between the number engaged in and the number dying in any given occupation, expressed as a rate per 1,000, is also fallacious. As we have already seen, the death-rate in the general population (page 101) varies greatly at different groups of ages. The death-rate among those engaged in any one trade or profession would similarly vary according to the relative number at the different ages engaged in it. In other words, it would depend on the *ages of the living*, which would vary in every occupation, (*a*) according as persons enter it early or late in life, and (*b*) according as the numbers that annually enter it increase or decrease. Dr. Farr, in his 14th Report gives the following example of the mistakes which would follow the adoption of this method. The death-rate of all farmers over 20 years of age is 28 per 1,000, of all tailors 20 in 1,000; but when tested by a comparison of the death-rate among men of corresponding ages, farmers are much healthier than tailors, as seen in the following table:—

Death-Rate per 1,000 *at Six Age-Groups of Farmers and Tailors.*

AGE.	25-	35-	45-	55-	65-	75-
Farmers . .	10·15	8·64	11·09	24·90	55·30	148·62
Tailors . .	11·63	14·15	16·74	28·18	76·47	155·28

(3) The only trustworthy method is to compare the mortality

of those engaged in one occupation, and of a given age, with the mortality of those engaged in another occupation *and of a corresponding age.*

(4) In some cases it is convenient to know the proportion of deaths furnished by different classes. Thus, in my Annual Report for Clapham (1886), the number of deaths occurring in the several social grades were classified as follows:—

	Number of Deaths.	Percentage of Total Deaths.
Nobility and Gentry	34	6·3
Professional Classes	80	14·8
Middle and Trading Classes	119	21·8
Industrial and Labouring Classes	312	57·1
All Classes	545	100·0

Of course in the absence of information as to the relative number of persons living in these different classes, we have no exact knowledge of their rate of mortality. Some indication of the relative healthiness of the classes may however be obtained by comparing the relative mortality from the chief zymotic diseases in each class. Thus, in the preceding instance, the industrial and labouring class furnished 57·1 per cent. of the total deaths, but 69 per cent. of the deaths from zymotic diseases. Where, as in the example quoted on page 151, the number of persons living and dying in each class is obtainable, most valuable results can be obtained. The fallacy connected with varying age distribution of the populations compared must in every case be borne in mind.

Dr. Ogle on Occupational Mortality.—In what follows on this subject, we shall follow very closely the important report of Dr. Ogle, in his Supplement to the 45th Annual Report of the Registrar-General, as this represents the most recent and trustworthy information on the subject, and the data on which it has been founded are more extensive than any previously employed. In Dr. Farr's supplement for 1851–60, the corresponding calculations were based upon the census numbers for 1861, and the deaths in 1860 and 1861; in his 1861–70 supplement, upon the census numbers for 1871, and the deaths in the same year. In Dr. Ogle's report, the deaths, in combination with ages and occupations, have been abstracted for three entire years, 1880–82. The inquiry was limited to males, because of the greater uncertainty attaching to statements of age and occupation in women. Males under 15 years of age were excluded, the influence of occupation below this age being inappreciable.

The number of *males aged fifteen years and upwards* at the 1881 census in England and Wales was 7,911,456, and the total deaths of males of these ages during the three years 1880–82 was 418,214. Dr. Ogle claims a high degree of trustworthiness for his results, on account of the width of his basis of observations and the precautions taken to insure uniformity in the abstraction of the statistics relating to the living and the dead. He points out, however, several causes of possible error.

Sources of Possible Error.—(1) Although the aggregate numbers both of the living and dead in these years are very great, the *numbers in individual trades*, and still more the numbers at each age-period, are, in many cases, but *small*. The amount of confidence in a series of observations is *ceteris paribus* proportional to the number of observations; and therefore for small trades or age-periods, where the numbers are few, the results must be received with hesitation.

(2) A more serious difficulty, already mentioned (p. 150), is the *vagueness with which the occupation may be returned*, both in the census and the death-registers, especially in the latter. Although the same clerks were employed in abstracting the two sets of returns, and uniformity of method was thus secured, the death returns are often more vague in regard to occupation than the census returns. To remedy this, and at the same time to widen the basis of operations, occupations likely to be confounded to any extent were grouped together. In some cases, even where the occupation was very definite, as that of a *coal-miner*, it was found necessary to do this, because, in many of the death-returns, coal-miners were not further specified than as *miners*. A geographical classification of miners was therefore adopted. Similarly, general and agricul-

tural labourers are often confused in the death-returns, and it was necessary, therefore, to group them together. In order to diminish the confusion between the two, the returns were given separately for ten selected counties in which the great mass of labour was agricultural.

(3) A still more serious difficulty is pointed out by Dr. Ogle, for which there appears to be no remedy, and which must always to some extent diminish the value of all calculations of the death-rate in different industries. Many trades, as that of a blacksmith or miner, require great muscular strength, and must be given up by persons who become weakly; and the latter may then raise the mortality of the lighter occupations to which they resort. Thus the death-rate of the more laborious occupations is unfairly lowered as compared with the death-rate (*a*) of those engaged in lighter occupations, or (*b*) of those who are returned as having no occupation, or (*c*) of those who have to betake themselves to odd jobs, as general labourers, messengers, costermongers and street-sellers.

(4) Another flaw in occupation death-rates, when taken as tests of relative healthiness, is the fact that those who follow the several industries do not start on equal terms as regards healthiness. A weakling will not become a navvy, but a shop man or tailor by preference. The occupations demanding grea muscular strength and activity, to some extent then, consist of picked men, stronger at the commencement, and maintained up to a certain standard by the fact that weaklings are drafted into lighter occupations.

After making full allowance for the preceding difficulties, the death-rates of different occupations still furnish most valuable indications of the relative salubrity of different occupations; and while small differences may be accidental, large differences must be taken as representing real differences of healthiness in the various occupations.

Mortality in Different Occupations.—Dr. Ogle gives, for each of about 400 occupations, the death-rate per 1,000 living at five age-periods: but of these the groups comprising the forty years between the 26th and 66th birthdays are the largest, and show the influence of occupation most markedly, and have been selected in the following table, compiled from Dr. Ogle's larger table. Before 25 the influence of occupation has not had time fully to develop, and after 65 the influence of retirement comes into play. In the first and second columns are given, for the sake of comparison, the corresponding mean annual death-rates, calculated from the data in Dr. Farr's two preceding decennial reports. It will be noticed that the death-rate at ages 25–45 in nearly every case has declined in the latter period 1880–1–2. In 65 of the 73 industries, for which the death-rates of the two periods are comparable, there is a reduction in this age-period; in one it is stationary, and in only 7 has it risen. In the second age-period (45–65) of the industries comparable, in only 35 has there been a fall, while in the remaining 38 the rate has risen. This is in strict accordance with the table on page 101, which shows that, independently of occupation, there has been a fall in the death-rate of males in the earlier, and some degree of rise in the later age-periods.

The fifth column, headed *Comparative Mortality Figure*, requires some explanation. There were during 1880–1–2, in England and Wales, 1,000 annual deaths per 64,641 males, aged 25–65, of whom 41,920 were under, and 22,721 were over, 45 years of age. The figures in this column are the number of deaths that would have occurred in the several occupations out of 64,641 males, distributed according to age, as in England and Wales. For instance, 41,920 of the clergy aged 25–45; and 22,721, aged 45–65, with a death-rate respectively of 4·64 and 15·93 per 1,000, gave 556 deaths. Thus the figure 556 represents the mean mortality of the clergy between 25 and 65, as compared with the mortality of all males of similar ages in England and Wales, which is 1,000.

The mortality figure for "all males" being 1,000, the death-rate of more than three-fifths of the industries is below this. The standard furnished by "all males," however, is a very unsatisfactory one, as it includes an enormous number permanently enfeebled in health and not engaged in any definite occupation.

Death-Rates of Males, 25–65 *years of age, in Different Occupations, in* 1860–1–1871, *and in* 1880–2; *and their Comparative Mortality Figures in* 1880–2.

Occupation.	Mean Annual Death-Rates per 1,000 living.				Comparative Mortality Figure, 1880-1-2.
	1860-1-1871.		1880-1-2.		
	Years of Age.		Years of Age.		Years of Age.
	25-45.	45-65.	25-45.	45-65.	25-65.
All Males	11·27	23·98	10·16	25.27	1000
Occupied Males	—	—	9·71	24·63	967
Unoccupied Males	—	—	32·43	36·20	2182
Males in Selected Healthy Districts	—	—	8·47	19·74	804
Clergyman, Priest, Minister	5·96	17·31	4 64	15·93	556
Gardener, Nurseryman	6·74	17 54	5·52	16 19	599
Farmer, Grazier	7·66	17·32	6·09	16·53	631
Labourer in Agricultural Counties	—	—	7·13	17·68	701
Schoolmaster, Teacher	9·82	23·56	6 41	19·98	719
Grocer	9·49	17·15	8·00	19·16	771
Fisherman	11·26	15·84	8·32	19·74	797
Carpenter, Joiner	9 44	21·36	7·77	21 74	820
Bookseller, Stationer	10·84	21·36	8·53	20·57	825
Barrister, Solicitor	9·87	22·97	7·54	23·13	842
Draper and Manchester Warehouseman	14·34	26·33	9·70	20·96	883
Groom, Domestic Coachman	—	—	8·53	23·28	887
Coal Miners (as represented by Miners in six districts)	—	—	7·64	25 11	891
Plasterer, Whitewasher	9·50	27·90	7·79	25 07	896
Watch and Clock Maker	10·78	24·90	9·26	22·64	903
Tanner, Fellmonger	10·43	26 57	7·97	25·37	911
Shoemaker	10·39	22·30	9 31	23·36	921
Artist, Engraver, Sculptor, Architect	11·73	22·91	8·39	25·07	921
Commercial Traveller	12·28	29·00	9·04	25·03	948
Corn Miller	9·32	26·65	8·40	26·62	957
Baker, Confectioner	10·72	26·39	8·70	26·12	958
Builder, Mason, Bricklayer	11·43	27·16	9·25	25·59	969
Blacksmith	10·07	23 88	9·29	25·67	973
Commercial Clerk and Insurance Service	14·28	28·88	10 48	24·49	996
Tobacconist	13·19	21·76	11·14	23·46	1000
Chemist, Druggist	13·92	23 56	10·58	25·16	1015
Tailor	12·92	24·79	10·73	26·47	1051
Printer	13·02	29·38	11·12	26·60	1071

Death-Rates of Males, 25–65 years of age, etc.—continued.

Occupation.	Mean Annual Death-Rates per 1,000 living. 1860-1-1871. Years of Age. 25–45.	45–65.	1880-1-2. Years of Age. 25–45.	45–65.	Comparative Mortality Figure, 1880-1-2. Years of Age. 25–65.
Wool, Worsted Manufacture (West Riding)	—	—	9·71	27·50	1032
Cotton, Linen Manufacture (Lancashire)	—	—	9·99	29·44	1088
Physician, Surgeon, General Practitioner	13·81	24·55	11·57	28·03	1122
Law Clerk	18·75	37·05	10·77	30·79	1151
Butcher	13·19	28·37	12·16	29·08	1170
Glass Manufacture	13·19	29·32	11·21	31·71	1190
Plumber, Painter, Glazier	12·48	34·66	11·07	32·49	1202
Cutler, Scissors, Needle, Saw, Tool-Maker	11·88	32·74	11·71	34·42	1273
Carter, Carrier, Haulier	—	—	12·52	33·00	1275
Bargeman, Lighterman, Waterman	14·99	30·78	14·25	31·13	1305
Musician, Music Master	18·94	34·76	13·78	32·39	1314
Hairdresser	15·11	30·10	13·64	33·25	1327
Brewer	19·26	36·86	13·90	34·25	1361
Cab, Omnibus, Service	15·94	35·28	15·39	36·83	1482
Chimney Sweep	17·53	42·87	13·73	41·54	1519
Innkeeper, Publican	18·01	34·14	18·02	33·68	1521
Messenger, Porter, Watchman	—	—	17·07	37·37	1565
File Maker	16·27	42·30	15·29	45·14	1667
Earthenware Manufacture	12·59	41·75	13·70	51·39	1742
Miner (Cornwall)	11·94	41·73	14·77	53·69	1839
Costermonger, Hawker, Street Seller	20·09	37·82	20·26	45·33	1879
General Labourer (London)	18·35	40·64	20·62	50·85	2020
Inn, Hotel, Servant	21·91	42·19	22·63	55·30	2205

Occupational Mortality Distributed as to Causes.—The preceding table gives the mortality *from all causes* in the several industries. To obtain the comparative mortality in each occupation from separate diseases or groups of diseases is an even more complicated task. It would form too gigantic a task to abstract all the deaths of males distributed as to ages, occupations and causes of death in combination; and samples of causes of death must be selected for each industry. Dr. Ogle gives a table founded on this basis in the same report (pages xxx.–xxxiii.). The minimum number of deaths with causes is fixed at 500, in order to constitute a sufficiently wide basis for calculations. Not only must the sample be large enough, but, as Dr. Ogle points out, it must be so extensively taken as to be free from peculiarities due to locality or season. We do not reproduce here Dr. Ogle's elaborate table founded on this basis, but in the following remarks shall incorporate some of its results.

Remarks on Special Occupations.—In the preceding table the occupations selected are given in the order of the lowness of their mortality, as shown by the comparative mortality figure.

The lowest mortality is enjoyed by the *Church* (556), and the mortality has fallen considerably since 1860–61–71, at both the two age-periods. *Schoolmasters* (719) are below *lawyers* (842), and still more below *doctors* (1,122) in mortality. This is probably due in part to the fact that the teachers in the public service (forming a great majority of the whole profession) have to undergo rigid medical examination before being admitted.

Gardeners are represented by a mortality figure of 599, farmers of 631, and agricultural labourers of 701. The higher mortality of labourers is largely due to their greater liability to phthisis and respiratory diseases. On the other hand, the *farmer* has a higher mortality under the headings of gout, alcoholism, and liver disease. There is some doubt in regard to *fishermen*, because of the possibility of some escaping both the census and death registration. Taking the figures as they stand, fishermen have a very low mortality from diseases of the nervous and respiratory systems and from phthisis, but a high mortality from accidents, rivalling coal-miners in this respect.

The figures as to *cabmen* (1,482), bargemen (1,305), carters (1,275), and costermongers (1,879), show that an open-air life in itself is not sufficient to ensure healthiness. Probably many engaged in these occupations have been driven to them by comparative unhealthiness. They also generally show a high mortality from alcoholic diseases, as well as from accident, phthisis, and respiratory diseases. *Commercial travellers* stand at 948, a considerable proportion of their mortality being due to intemperance.

Brewers (1,361), *innkeepers* (1,521), and *inn-servants* (2,205) have an excessive mortality which is chiefly due to alcoholism. For innkeepers and publicans the mortality from alcoholism is more than five times higher than the average, and from liver diseases is six times as high as the average. They also show the highest mortality from gout and from urinary diseases, with the exception of occupations dealing with lead. Spite of these high figures, a large proportion of both publicans and brewers must be of temperate habits, for the comparative mortality figure for recognised intemperate persons is, according to Mr. Neison's data, 3,240.

There is a decline in the mortality of all the following *shop-keepers*, the comparative mortality of which is now for coal-merchant, 758; grocer, 771; stationer and bookseller, 825; general shopkeeper, 865; draper, 883; ironmonger, 895; fish-monger, 974; tobacconist, 1,000; milk-butter-cheesemonger, 1009; chemist, 1,015; greengrocer, 1,015. Grocers suffer much less than drapers from phthisis and respiratory diseases, especially the former; but more from circulatory diseases, and slightly more from alcoholism and suicide. The mortality of grocers from phthisis is one of the lowest, that of drapers one of the highest.

Butchers have a high mortality (1,170), which is largely due to excessive indulgence; their mortality from alcoholism, liver diseases and urinary diseases, respectively, being almost identical with that of brewers. Like other trades in which there is evidence of alcoholic excess, their mortality is high from phthisis (the figure being 261 against an average of 220 for all males).

The mortality figure of *bakers* and confectioners is 958, almost the same as that of millers. Their mortality from alcoholism and suicide is very high, but phthisis is hardly above the average, notwithstanding their exposure to dust.

Hatters (1,064) are subjected to great alternations of temperature, and, like hairdressers (1,327), have a high mortality from phthisis and from the effects of alcoholism.

For both *tailors* (1,051) and *shoemakers* (921) the mortality must be regarded as high. Their mortality from phthisis and from diseases of the circulatory and nervous systems is high, as well as from alcoholism and suicide.

Printers (1,071) and bookbinders (1,167) have both a high mortality. The high mortality of printers is entirely due to phthisis (461 against 220 for all males). Except costermongers, and occupations subject to dust inhalations, no mortality from phthisis approaches that of printers. The mortality of printers from lead poisoning, even if renal and nervous diseases be included, is but slight.

The *earthenware and china manufacture* was noted by Dr. Farr in 1871 as one of the unhealthiest trades in this country. Now its mortality figure is 1,742, which is only exceeded by costermongers, Cornish miners, and inn and hotel servants. This excessive mortality is chiefly from phthisis and respiratory diseases (1,118 as against 402 for all males). Only in one occupation, that of Cornish miners, is the mortality from these two causes higher. Circulatory diseases also rank very high, the "potter's asthma" in turn giving rise to cardiac disease.

In the textile manufactures there appears to be a gradation in mortality, probably connected with the amount of dust and the temperature in each process, from cotton manufacture, 1088; woollen and worsted, 1032; carpet manufacture, 945; silk, 845; lace, 755; to hosiery manufacture, 717.

	All Males.	Cotton Manufacture.	Woollen.	Hosiery.
Total Mortality Figure . .	1,000	1,088	1,032	717
Mortality Figure for Phthisis and Respiratory Diseases	402	543	462	283

Plumbers have a high mortality (1,202), which is mainly determined by lead-poisoning, though alcoholism and accident also range high. The mortality figure under lead-poisoning is 21, the highest for any occupation except that for filemakers. It would probably be higher, were it practicable to take painters separately. The mortality figure from urinary diseases is 100, only exceeded by filemakers. Gout and diseases of the nervous and circulatory systems also range very high. As early as 1854, Garrod found that 30 per cent. of his hospital patients with gout had been subjected to lead-poisoning.

Cutlers (1,309) and filemakers (1,667) each inhale metallic dust mixed with stone-dust. The mortality figure for cutlers from phthisis and respiratory diseases is 760, for filemakers 782. *Filemakers* are also exposed to lead-poisoning, caused by the use of a cushion of lead on which to strike their files, their comparative mortality figure from plumbism being 41, as compared with 21 for plumbers and painters.

Miners constitute an important portion of the industrial community, as 1 in every 19 males between 25 and 65 is a miner. Owing to the unfortunate fact that the death-returns commonly do not distinguish between the different kinds of miners, it is impracticable to estimate separately the mortality of each kind of miners. At least one-fifth of the mortality of all miners is due to accident. In the following statements from Dr. Ogle's report a geographical classification has been adopted, which roughly differentiates the nature of the mineral in which miners work. *Coal-miners*, as thus distinguished, have a surprisingly low mortality, except in South Wales, where it is slightly higher than for all males in the same district; and even here the low mortality would be maintained if accidents were excluded. If accidents were excluded for all miners, they would have a mortality only slightly higher than that for all agriculturists (farmers, agricultural labourers, and gardeners). It must be remembered, however, that coal-miners are a picked body of men, while the general population comprises numerous sick and weakly ones. But even when compared with quarrymen or blacksmiths, who must be picked in the same sense, the mortality of coal-miners, excluding accident, is low. Coal-miners have an appalling mortality from accident, only approached by other forms of mining, stone and slate quarrying, and fishing. Nearly one-half of the accidental deaths were from the falling in of the sides or roofs of mines, and one-fourth by fire-damp or by choke-damp. Under other headings they are below the average, except for respiratory diseases, for which they stand at 202 as against 182 for all males in England and Wales. Probably many cases of so-called "miner's phthisis" should come under this head; though, even allowing these to stand as at present, the figure for phthisis among coal-miners is only 126. Coal-dust is comparatively free from sharp angles, and does not therefore cause such irritation of the lungs as metallic dust. English, Belgian, and German evidence all shows a comparative immunity of coal-miners from phthisis, and it has been supposed that coal-dust possesses some inhibitory power on the development of tubercles. Partly owing to the fact that there is some doubt whether "miner's phthisis" is tubercular or bronchitic in character, it is still however dubious whether the low mortality of coal-miners from phthisis is a part of their general healthiness and exemption from disease of all kinds, or whether coal-miners possess some special immunity from phthisis.

Among *Cornish miners* the mortality figure is 1,839 as compared with 887 for all Cornish males, having considerably increased since Dr. Farr's last report on the subject for 1861–70. This increase is probably due in part to emigration of the more robust, consequent on the decadence of the industry, just the opposite of what happens in other mining districts; but this does not entirely explain why mining in Cornwall is apparently so much more unhealthy than elsewhere. The great bulk of the excessive mortality among Cornish miners is from phthisis and respiratory disease, which stand at 1,148 as against 368 for all Cornish males, and 459 for the miners of South Wales and Monmouthshire.

Chimney sweeps have a mortality figure of 1,519, and an excessive mortality under nearly all the chief headings. Their liability to cancer appears to be eight times as great as that of all males.

We may summarize, in conclusion, some of the most important facts bearing on the influence of foul air, of dust, alcoholic excess, and lead-poisoning on the health of those exposed to their effects. The following tables given by Dr. Ogle will illustrate these points.

Comparative Mortality of Males working in Air of Different Degrees of Purity, from Phthisis and Diseases of the Respiratory Organs.

	Phthisis.	Diseases of Respiratory System.	The two together.
Fishermen	108	90	198
Agriculturists	115	122	237
Grocers	167	116	283
Drapers	301	129	430
Tailors	285	186	471
Printers	461	166	627

Comparative Mortality of Males in Certain Dust-Inhaling Occupations from Phthisis and Diseases of the Respiratory Organs.

	Comparative Mortality Figure (1880-1-2) that of all Males being 1000.	Phthisis.	Diseases of Respiratory Organs.	The two together.
Coal Miner	891	126	202	328
Carpenter, Joiner	820	204	133	337
Baker, Confectioner	958	212	186	398
Mason, Builder, Bricklayer.	969	252	201	453
Wool Manufacture.	1032	257	205	462
Cotton Manufacture	1088	272	271	543
Quarryman	1122	308	274	582
Cutler	1309	371	389	760
Filemaker	1667	433	350	783
Earthenware Manufacture	1742	473	645	1,118
Cornish Miner	1839	690	458	1,148
Fishermen		108	90	198

Fishermen form, in the preceding tables, a convenient standard of comparison, as they have no exposure to dust, and enjoy a pure atmosphere for their work. It will be seen that the dust from textile fabrics is much more dangerous than that from coal or wood or flour, while the dust of stone and metals is still more deleterious. The high mortality among Cornish miners and pottery makers is due in part to their working in confined spaces, and consequently inhaling the stone-dust in much larger amount.

The following table from Dr. Farr's Supplement to the Registrar-General's 35th Annual Report illustrates very strikingly the effect of tippling on the death-rate at different age-groups:—

Annual Death-Rates per 1,000 *at Four Ages among Clergymen and Protestant Ministers, and among Publicans and Wine Merchants.*

Ages.	Clergymen.	Protestant Ministers.	Publicans, Beer-Sellers, Wine & Spirit Merchants.
25–35	4·65	5·83	14·49
35–45	6·28	7·30	20·44
45–55	13·24	9·33	28·50
55–65	22·70	24·60	43·03

Dr. Ogle's figures for 1871–80 show that the mortality from liver diseases (perhaps the most trustworthy test of alcoholic excess) is six times as high among innkeepers and publicans, and two and a half times as high among brewers, as among the generality of males. In occupations where alcoholic excess is common, the mortality from gout, urinary and nervous diseases, and from suicide, is also invariably high; and alcoholism likewise contributes to the mortality from phthisis.

Lead-poisoning is evidenced in four occupations—viz., printers, earthenware makers, painters with plumbers and glaziers, and filemakers; though it prevails to a considerable extent only in the two latter. These two show also an extremely high mortality from renal diseases, confirming the general medical opinion that lead-poisoning causes renal disease. In the four years 1879–82, only 229 deaths of males were ascribed to lead-poisoning, though this number would doubtless be greatly increased were it possible to include the deaths from renal nervous and other affections produced by lead-poisoning. The 229 deaths were distributed as follows:—

House Painter	91	Iron Moulder	2
Plumber	28	Calico Printer, dyer	2
Earthenware Maker	16	Paint, Colour-maker	2
File-Cutter	14	Glazier	1
Lead (? White Lead) Worker	8	Artist	1
Printer	6	Lead Roller	1
Lead Miner	3	Lead Mine Agent	1
Gas Fitter	3	Caulker	1
Coach Painter	3	Children (under 15)	6
Whitesmith	2	Others	36
Glass Cutter	2		

The annual death-rates from lead-poisoning among males over fifteen years of age, as deduced from a comparison of these figures with the census returns of 1881, are as follows. Reliance cannot, however, be placed on rates calculated from so few data:—

Filemaker	466 per million living.
Painter, Plumber, Glazier	224 ,, ,, ,,
Earthenware Maker	152 ,, ,, ,,
Gas Fitter	62 ,, ,, ,,
Printer	27 ,, ,, ,,
All other males	4 ,, ,, ,,

For further details on all the questions discussed in this chapter, which have a great practical importance, the reader is referred to Dr. Ogle's invaluable report, pages xxi.–lxiv., which ought to do much to stimulate preventive measures in the case of unhealthy occupations.

CHAPTER XI.

MORTALITY FROM ZYMOTIC DISEASES.

Methods of Estimating.—Zymotic Death-rate.—Measles.—Scarlet Fever.—Case Mortality.—Relation of Scarlet Fever to Age and Sex.—Geographical Distribution of Scarlet Fever and Diphtheria.—Diphtheria.—Whooping Cough.—Fever.—Enteric and Typhus Fever.—Diarrhœa.

WE have in the preceding chapters shown the effect produced by various social and other conditions on the general mortality. In the next place we must consider the mortality from individual diseases and from groups of diseases. In the first place, as to the **methods of stating** this mortality. This will vary according to the object in view. (1) The first plan, useful only for purely medical purposes, consists in stating the *proportion of deaths to persons attacked* with any given disease. This method is of importance to medical men, as from the results thus obtained deductions are drawn concerning the effect of a particular line of treatment. We may point out the liability of this method to error before passing on to the methods of statement usually adopted by vital statisticians.

(*a*) The number of facts manipulated is often so small as not to warrant exact conclusions. I have recently investigated an outbreak of enteric fever due to infected milk, in which 21 cases occurred. Of these 15 were treated either at home or in a public hospital, while 6 were treated in another public hospital. Of the first 15 cases none died, while 2 of the last 6 were fatal. The difference in fatality was almost certainly due to accidental causes, and any inferences as to skill of treatment would be altogether fallacious. Speaking generally, therapeutical results or etiological theories, advanced on the strength of *percentages from a small number of cases, must be accepted with caution.*

(*b*) The two groups compared may have a different age and sex constitution, and it is a notorious fact that the death-rate from nearly all diseases is largely influenced by these factors, and especially by age. This is seen in the following table from Murchison on Continued Fevers.

Mortality per cent. of Males and Females Attacked at Different Ages.

Age.		0-5.	5-10.	10-15.	15-20.	20-25.	25-30.	30-35.	35-40.	40-45.	45-50.
Typhus Fever	Males	12·50	11·17	11·12	12·76	23·30	17·17	32·69	26·04	28·12	33·33
	Females	12·06	11·28	12·86	15·48	20·36	20·50	25·59	26·36	26·61	21·87
Enteric Fever	Males	8·03	2·24	1·60	4·65	11·04	17·66	20·60	31·57	33·58	45·32
	Females	6·69	3·59	2·28	4·46	10·33	15·17	20·55	25·92	30·79	42·54

Of course, by splitting up the deaths at all ages into groups at different ages, the number of individual facts at each age is reduced, and thus the fallacy due to paucity of data is introduced. This, however, is preferable to the lumping together of two sets of facts which are not comparable with each other. In stating percentages *the number of facts on which they are founded should always be given*, as their trustworthiness can then be gauged.

(*c*) In the case of infectious diseases, the character of the particular epidemic must be taken into account. One epidemic of diphtheria may differ in virulence from another, and comparison between methods of treatment in the two epidemics would be consequently largely vitiated. Similarly, it would be unfair to compare the treatment at the beginning of an outbreak of cholera, when 50 per cent. of those attacked usually die, with the treatment in the later and milder period of the epidemic.

(2) The mortality from any given disease or group of diseases may be stated as *a proportion to the deaths from all causes.* This method is, however, essentially fallacious, as it constitutes a ratio between two factors, of which both are variable, viz., the mortality from the specified disease, and the mortality from all causes. Dr. Ransome gives the following example of its fallacious character. Suppose a town of 100,000 with 2,000 annual deaths, of which 500 are caused by phthisis. Here the general death-rate is 20 per 1,000; the death-rate from phthisis is 5 per 1,000 living, and the proportion of deaths from phthisis to the total deaths is 250 to 1,000. In another town having the same population the total deaths are 4,000, and therefore the death-rate 40 per 1,000 inhabitants; the deaths from phthisis are 1,000, and therefore the death-rate from phthisis is 10 per 1,000; but the proportion of the phthisical to the total mortality is 250 to 1,000, as before. In the second town, therefore, there is by the latter test apparently no worse condition, so far as phthisis is concerned, than in the first, though matters are really twice as bad.

The following table, abstracted from the local report of a medical officer of health, gives another instance of this fallacious method:—

	1879.	1880.	1881.	1882.	1883.	1886.
Zymotic Death-Rate per 1,000 Inhabitants	4·14	3·35	2·71	3·72	2·57	3·58
General Death-Rate per 1,000	20·56	17·67	17·97	18·70	16·71	22·33
Percentage of Deaths from Zymotic Diseases to Deaths from All Causes	17·8	16·1	13·6	17·2	11·4	15·3

The zymotic and general death-rates are in this table accurate indications of mortality; but if the two first columns are compared, it will be seen that the proportion between the two gives no indication as to their relative mortality. Such relative mortality might be increased either by a diminution in total deaths or an increase in zymotic deaths, though the inference to be drawn in the two cases would be very different.

For large communities, or for the whole country, when fallacies due to varying age and sex constitution can be eliminated, it is often convenient to know the percentage of deaths due to different causes. The following table shows the percentage of deaths from different groups of diseases in England and Wales during 1886; and in a parallel column the rate of mortality per million of the population.

Deaths in England and Wales in 1886.

Causes of Death.	Number of Deaths.	Percentage of Total Deaths.	Death-Rate per Million Living.
Zymotic Diseases	73,747	13·7	2,648
Parasitic Diseases	990	0·2	35
Dietetic Diseases	1,656	0·3	59
Constitutional Diseases	92,751	17·3	3,330
Developmental Diseases	45,103	8·4	1,618
Local Diseases	276,302	51·4	9,915
Violence	17,444	3·2	626
Ill-defined and not Specified Causes	29,283	5·5	1,047
	537,276	100·	19,278

In the following table some of the more important diseases are treated separately, the death-rate per million living and the percentage of total deaths being given for each.

Deaths in England and Wales in 1886.

Causes of Death.	Number of Deaths.	Percentage of Total Deaths.	Death-Rate per Million Living.
Smallpox	275	·05	10
Measles	12,013	2·24	431
Scarlet Fever	5,986	1·11	215
Diphtheria	4,098	·76	147
Whooping Cough	12,936	2·41	464
Fever (Typhus, Typhoid, and Ill-defined)	5,911	1·10	213
Diarrhœal Diseases	25,284	4·76	907
Puerperal Fever and Diseases of Childbirth	3,877	·72	140
Cancer	16,243	3·02	583
Phthisis	47,872	8·91	1,718
Other Tubercular Diseases	20,203	3·76	726
Diseases of Nervous System (including convulsions)	74,017	13·78	2,656
Diseases of Circulatory System	45,332	8·44	1,625
Diseases of Respiratory System (including Croup)	103,892	19·33	3,594
Diseases of Digestive System	31,733	5·91	1,140
Diseases of Urinary System	12,394	2·30	445
Violence	17,444	3·25	626
Ill-defined and not Specified	29,283	5·45	1,047
Other Causes of Death	68,483	12·74	—
Total Deaths	537,276	100·	19,278

(3) *The deaths from each individual case should be stated per thousand or per million of the entire population.* These death-rates are shown for the more important diseases during the decennium 1871–80 in the following diagram, the mortality of males and females being distinguished by a continuous line in the case of males, and a dotted line in the case of females.

CHART SHOWING RELATIVE MORTALITY FROM SEVERAL DISEASES PER MILLION LIVING IN DECENNIUM, 1871-80.

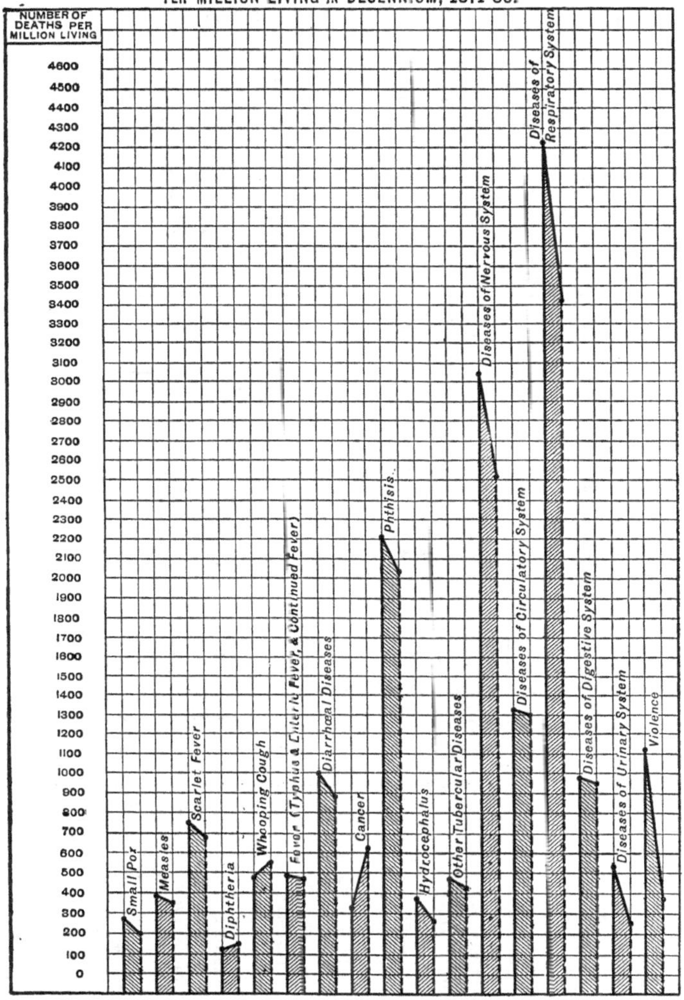

In the following table the mortality per million from the more important causes is given for successive years and groups of years.

Annual Mortality from Several Causes per Million Living at all Ages in Successive Periods and Years.

	1851–60.	1861–70.	1871–80.	1881.	1882.	1883.	1884.	1885.	1886.	1887.
All Causes	22,165	22,416	21,272	18,880	19,560	19,536	19,511	19,010	19,278	18,790
Small-Pox	221	163	236	119	50	36	82	103	10	18
Measles	412	440	378	280	481	348	416	526	431	594
Scarlet Fever	876	972	716	548	520	472	399	231	215	278
Diphtheria	109	185	121	121	151	158	185	163	147	157
Whooping Cough	503	527	512	416	577	391	422	477	464	398
Fever — including Typhus				21	36	33	12	12	9	7
Fever — including Enteric	908	885	484	212	229	227	234	173	182	182
Fever — including Ill-defined				44	38	36	28	24	22	18
Puerperal Fever and	164	165	167	88	98	98	91	88	75	87
Diseases of Childbirth				74	74	71	69	74	65	61
Diarrhœal Diseases	1,080	1,076	935	570	664	610	1,001	498	907	733
Cancer	317	387	473	520	532	546	559	566	583	606
Phthisis	2,679	2,475	2,116	1,825	1,844	1,870	1,812	1,752	1,718	1,591
Hydrocephalus	397	347	317	705	729	707	738	654	726	658
Other Tubercular Diseases	407	437	445							
Diseases of Nervous System (including Convulsions)	2,741	2,785	2,770	2,600	2,644	2,702	2,657	2,604	2,656	2,546
Diseases of Circulatory System and Dropsy	1,247	1,349	1,477	1,369	1,372	1,465	1,495	1,579	1,625	1,643
Diseases of Respiratory System	3,021	3,364	3,760	3,427	3,555	3,656	3,317	3,699	3,594	3,572
Diseases of Digestive System	1,004	981	978	1,103	1,121	1,117	1,135	1,083	1,140	1,068
Diseases of Urinary System	214	298	392	381	394	446	438	441	445	439
Violence	733	765	733	697	669	675	651	625	626	642

The figures in the above table can be easily converted into rates per thousand by inserting a decimal point at the third place to the left.

Zymotic Death-Rate.—The term *Zymotic* was introduced by Dr. Farr, and it is practically so convenient that we propose to adhere to it, although *Specific Febrile Diseases* would be a more correct designation. The diseases comprised under this head are enumerated at page 26. They have such a varied origin that a rate compounded of all these would be of but secondary importance. The Registrar-General, however, gives the **death-rate from the seven chief infectious diseases** (small-pox, measles, scarlet fever, diphtheria, whooping cough, fever, and diarrhœa), and this is usually described as the zymotic death-rate. As a test of sanitary condition, this rate possesses considerable value, which must not, however, be exaggerated. To begin with, the prevalence of such diseases varies greatly in different districts, according to the proportional number of young children in each, apart altogether from any differences in sanitary condition. Then again, although whooping cough

Death-Rate per 1,000 *Living from Each of the Seven Chief Zymotic Diseases in England and Wales.*

	1851–60.	1861–70.	1871–80.	1881.	1882.	1883.	1884.	1885.	1886.	1887.
Small-Pox	·221	·163	·236	·119	·050	·036	·032	·103	·010	·018
Measles	·412	·440	·378	·280	·481	·348	·416	·526	·431	·594
Scarlet Fever	·876	·972	·716	·548	·520	·472	·309	·231	·215	·278
Diphtheria	·109	·185	·121	·121	·151	·158	·135	·163	·147	·157
Whooping Cough . .	·503	·527	·512	·416	·577	·391	·422	·477	·464	·398
Fever { Typhus Fever				·021	·036	·033	·012	·012	·009	·007
Fever { Enteric ,,	·908	·885	·484	·212	·229	·227	·234	·173	·182	·182
Fever { Continued ,,				·044	·038	·036	·028	·024	·022	·018
Diarrhœal Diseases . .	1·080	1·076	·935	·570	·664	·610	1·001	·498	·907	·733
Death-Rate from Seven Chief Infectious Diseases . . .	4·109	4·248	3·382	2·331	2·746	2·311	2·779	2·207	2·387	2·385

and measles have a much greater effect in increasing the mortality than diphtheria and enteric fever, they are much less amenable to sanitary measures than the latter diseases. An accumulation of children unprotected by a previous attack of the two first of these diseases, along with a spell of severe weather, might cause a great increase of zymotic mortality in any given locality, without its being of necessity in a less sanitary condition than another which had escaped. Notwithstanding these objections, the zymotic death-rate gives approximate indications, and it can easily be separated into its component parts, as in the preceding table.

Measles.—In stating annually the mortality from some of the infectious diseases, it should be remembered that their infrequent appearance in the death-returns may be caused by the fact that there are but few in the population who have not purchased immunity by a previous attack. After a large epidemic of measles, or whooping cough, or scarlet fever, there is generally a lull for several years. Dr. Ransome has investigated the influence of what he calls *cyclical waves*, which appear to be independent of the accumulation of unprotected persons. From the Swedish Tables of Mortality (Epidemiological Society Transactions, 1881–82) he has constructed charts, which show that, in the case of scarlet fever, there is not only a short cycle of from four to six years, but also a long undulation of from 15 to 20 years or more, "which may be likened to a vast wave of disease upon which the lesser epidemics show like ripples upon the surface of an ocean swell."

The chief undulations of the measles curve seem to rise with fall of temperature, and *vice versâ*; and whooping cough seems to be influenced by much the same conditions. Humidity of air seems to favour mortality from measles much more than from whooping cough (Ransome).

An examination of the London weekly returns of mortality from 1840–84 proves that in the Metropolis there are two distinct seasons of the year in which the prevalence of measles, as measured by deaths, is above the general level of the year, one period having its maximum in May and June, and the other in November, December, and early January, the winter period being the more considerable (Registrar-General's Report, 1884).

Monthly Distribution of Deaths from Measles per 1,200 *in the Year.*

	London, 1840-84.	Berlin, 1875-83.	Bradford, Birmingham, Bristol, Brighton, Wolverhampton, 1871-84.	Lancashire Towns, 1871-84.
January . . .	111	51	92	116
February . . .	80	56	73	91
March . . .	88	65	105	107
April	102	92	134	135
May	110	185	136	120
June	118	240	136	123
July	105	202	94	101
August . . .	89	78	87	74
September . .	66	44	47	49
October . . .	79	36	74	73
November . .	112	69	90	90
December . .	140	82	132	121
	1,200	1,200	1,200	1,200

It will be seen from the preceding table that the winter excess in other places than London is nearly absent. All these towns or groups of towns show an excess of measles from April to July, and have a minimum in the autumn—usually in September or October; but the winter excess, which occurs in London, is hardly appreciable in the other towns. On the whole, it seems probable, "though the statement must be made with some reserve, that when the measles mortality in a town is habitually high, there are in it two measles seasons—a summer and a winter season; and that when the measles mortality is habitually low, the winter prevalence is either absent or comparatively slight."

Death-Rate per 1,000 *from Measles in Different Populations.*

	1882.	1883.	1884.	1885.	1886.	1887.
England and Wales . . .	0·48	0·35	0·42	0·52	0·41	0·59
London	0·60	0·62	0·55	0·72	0·50	0·69
28 Great English Towns . .	0·67	0·50	0·60	0·69	0·54	0·79
50 other Towns	0·58	0·41	0·45	0·75	0·52	0·54
Rural Districts	0·33	0·23	0·28	0·37	0·33	0·46

Scarlet Fever.—The following table shows the mortality from scarlet fever in different districts and years.

Death-Rate per 1,000 *from Scarlet Fever in Different Populations.*

	1882.	1883.	1884.	1885.	1886.	1887.
England and Wales . . .	0·52	0·47	0·40	0·23	0·21	0·27
London	0·52	0·51	0·36	0·17	0·17	0·34
28 Great English Towns . .	0·55	0·57	0·45	0·24	0·25	0·39
50 other Towns	0·65	0·55	0·51	0·25	0·26	0 25
Rural Districts	0·47	0·39	0·34	0·21	0·18	0 21

From 1882 to the end of 1886 there was a progressive decline in scarlet fever mortality in this country; but in 1887 an abrupt and general rise occurred, the mortality being nearly 29 per cent. higher than in 1886. In London the mortality from scarlet fever was twice as high as in the two preceding years, though it was 28 per cent. below the decennial average, which was 0·47 per 1,000 persons. Spite of this, however, there was, during the autumn and winter of 1887, considerable alarm in London, arising in part from the strain on the accommodation provided by the Metropolitan Asylums Board Hospitals for scarlet fever. This strain was doubtless due in part to the increased prevalence of scarlet fever, but also largely to the fact that there is an increased willingness to enter these hospitals. The larger use of hospitals is shown by the increased proportion borne by deaths in hospital to external deaths. In 1878 the deaths in the London Fever Hospital and the Asylums

Board Hospitals were only 7 per cent. of the whole mortality from scarlet fever in London; in 1879–82 they were 9–11 per cent.; in 1883 they rose to 13·2 per cent.; in 1884 to 17·6, in 1885 to 20·2, in 1886 to 22·7, and finally, in 1887, to 33·6 per cent. of the total deaths. If we assume the proportion of cases to deaths (case mortality) in hospitals to represent the proportion for the whole of London, then the number of cases of scarlet fever in London during the last eight years was as follows:—

1880	28,039 cases.
1881	21,376 „
1882	23,194 „
1883	18,748 „
1884	13,912 „
1885	8,886 „
1886	8,185 „
1887	13,841 „

The deaths from scarlet fever in London during 1887 numbered 1,447, while those from measles during the same period numbered 2,894, and yet no alarm appears to have been felt in regard to the latter disease.

Relation of Mortality to Prevalence of Scarlet Fever.—We cannot assume that the mortality holding good in one outbreak will be maintained in others. In the previous calculation of the number of scarlet fever cases in London during 1880–87 the mortality has been obtained *separately for each outbreak* as the result of hospital experience. The hospital cases probably represent a graver portion of each outbreak; and if this be so, the total number of cases in the foregoing calculation has been under-estimated. The reports of the London Fever Hospital and Metropolitan Asylums Board Hospitals show that in 1875–80 the death-rate from scarlet fever was 120 per 1,000 cases; in 1881–85, 96 per 1,000 cases; and in one of these years, 1881, only 81 per 1,000. It may be argued, therefore, that a diminished mortality from scarlet fever implies either a correspondingly diminished prevalence of the disease, or only that a milder type of the disease now occurs.

N

If the former supposition is correct, then we have reason to fear recurrences of scarlet fever more extensively, as an accumulation of unprotected persons occurs.

Relation of Scarlet Fever to Age and Sex.—The following table is based on nearly half a million deaths from scarlet fever, which have been registered in England and Wales in the 27 years, 1859–85 (49th Annual Report of Registrar-General, 1886).

Mean Annual Mortality from Scarlet Fever per Million Living at Successive Age-Periods, 1859–85.

Age.	Annual Deaths per Million Living.	
	Males.	Females.
0–1	1,664	1,384
1–2	4,170	3,874
2–3	4,676	4,491
3–4	4,484	4,332
4–5	3,642	3,556
0–5	3,681	3,482
5–10	1,667	1,613
10–15	346	381
15–20	111	113
20–25	59	77
25–35	36	58
35 and upwards	13	15
All Ages.	778	717

It will be seen that in each sex the mortality from scarlet fever rises to a maximum in the third year of life, and then falls, at first slowly, but afterwards rapidly, becoming smaller at each successive age-period. In the first ten years of life, in which there is the greatest number of deaths, the male is considerably higher than the female mortality, though afterwards their relative position is reversed.

The large basis on which the above rates are calculated

renders it certain that the differences above shown between the two sexes and different ages are not accidental or transitory. The question then arises, Are the differences due to *differences of prevalence* or *differences of case mortality?* In answering this question, the Registrar-General's Report for 1886 gives the following table. It embodies the facts as to age, sex, and result of 17,795 cases of scarlet fever in the metropolitan fever hospitals during the twelve years 1874–85; and in addition the official reports for Christiania, in Norway, of 5,000 cases which occurred there in 1870–72. It was necessary to include these because the returns of the London hospitals do not differentiate each year of the 0–5 period, during which the prevalence of scarlet fever is at its maximum. As the case mortality in Christiania for the aggregate 0–5 period was nearly the same as that of the corresponding period in London, it may fairly be assumed that the rates for individual years were likewise similar.

Case Mortality.—Deaths per 1,000 *Cases of Scarlet Fever in Hospitals*, 1874–85.

Age.	Males.	Females.
0–1	395	442
1–2	384	343
2–3	255	226
3–4	184	174
4–5	130	112
0–5	241	217
5–10	106	97
10–15	56	53
15–20	40	34
20–25	39	32
25–35	75	43
35 and upwards	85	65

These figures are very striking, and show that age and sex have much greater influence on prognosis than is generally acknowledged. Males are in greater danger when attacked than females; but the difference due to sex is as nothing in comparison with that due to age, shown in the table.

It will be seen by a comparative view of the two preceding tables that the prevalence of scarlet fever (as indicated by its mortality) and the case mortality rapidly diminish as age advances, though the case mortality begins to increase again after the age of twenty-five. The general result of the preceding facts is, that the longer an attack is deferred the less likely is it to occur at all; and that even if it occur eventually, the less likely is it to end fatally.

Geographical Distribution of Scarlet Fever and Diphtheria. —During the year 1884 (47th Annual Report of Registrar-General), of the 44 registration counties, there were 18 in which the death-rate from diphtheria in 1884 was above the rate for the whole of England and Wales; in 11 of the 18 there was the same excess in the three previous years; and in 9 of these 11 the rate was also above the average for the decennium 1871-80. The counties which are thus shown to be much more liable to diphtheria than others form two tolerably definite areas, "one having its base in the south-eastern counties—Sussex, Hampshire, Surrey, and Kent, and stretching upwards along the eastern side of England through Middlesex, Hertfordshire, Essex, Cambridgeshire and Bedfordshire, occasionally reaching Norfolk, Nottinghamshire, and Lincolnshire; and the other area, having its nucleus in North Wales and Shropshire, and tending to spread through Herefordshire and other bordering counties, as also in some years into South Wales, Monmouthshire, and even across the Bristol Channel into Somersetshire."

Thus diphtheria was comparatively absent from the northern counties. But in these very counties the scarlet fever rate was highest in 1884; and although the geographical distribution of scarlet fever does not seem to be so constant as that of diphtheria, it is generally commonest in mining and manufacturing counties. In these counties there is a large proportion of young children; and as scarlet fever, like diphtheria, is a disease which specially affects children, some correction must be made on this account. In regard to diphtheria, which prevails in counties where there is not a large proportion of children, such correction would tend to increase the contrast. But in regard to scarlet fever age-distribution must be taken into account. If we confine our attention to the scarlet fever occurring during the 0–5 age-period, when the disease is most fatal, it is still found that scarlet fever is most destructive in the industrial and mining districts.

Diphtheria.—The returns under the heading of diphtheria cannot be regarded as trustworthy, owing to the confusion with croup and other diseases. In the Registrar-General's returns all deaths are returned under this head which are distinctly designated on the certificate as diphtheria, or as *cynanche maligna*, or malignant sore throat. But many deaths from diphtheria are returned as ulcerated throat, quinsy, croup, laryngitis, or membranous laryngitis, and these appear under other heads.

The mortality from diphtheria in 1887 for England and Wales was 150 per million of the population. At p. 172 is shown the corresponding mortality for a series of years. During 1887 in London 961 deaths were ascribed to diphtheria, or 180 in excess of the decennial average, after due correction for growth of population. This excess may possibly be due in part to the diminution of deaths returned as croup; but even taking diphtheria and croup together, there is still an excess of 58 deaths over the decennial average. "Be the explanation what it may, the registered mortality from diphtheria has been considerably higher in each of the last six years, 1882–87, than in any previous year since 1864, while during the six years themselves it has remained almost constant, the rate per 1,000 varying only from 0·21 to 0·24." (Annual Summary, 1887.)

It will be convenient to compare the rates of mortality in the 28 great towns with the rates of sickness in 41 compulsory notification towns for scarlet fever and diphtheria at this point (see also page 40).

Sickness and Death-Rates per 1,000 of the Population in Large Towns from Scarlet Fever and Diphtheria.

		1883.	1884.	1885.	1886.	1887.
Diphtheria	Sickness-Rate	0·33	0·39	0·36	0·36	0·46
	Death-Rate	0·158	0·185	0·163	0·147	0·18
Scarlet Fever	Sickness-Rate	3·59	3·81	4·64	4·12	6·90
	Death-Rate	0·57	0·45	0·24	0·25	0·39

Whooping Cough.—The prevalence of whooping cough in a series of years is shown in the table on page 172. In the decennium 1871–80, there was nearly the same incidence, as indicated by mortality, as in 1861–70. It appears to be a disease but little amenable to sanitary precautions, one reason of this being that it occurs at a very early age, and there is consequent difficulty in separating the sick from the healthy. The relative mortality from whooping cough in different groups of places is shown in the following table :—

Death-Rate per 1,000 from Whooping Cough in Different Populations.

	1882.	1883.	1884.	1885.	1886.	1887.
England and Wales	0·58	0·39	0·42	0·44	0·44	0·39
London	1·20	0·40	0·79	0·61	0·68	0·70
28 Great Towns. .	0·90	0·46	0·64	0·60	0·54	0·62
50 Other Towns .	0·47	0·37	0·33	0·53	0·42	0·33
Rural Districts . .	0·37	0·32	0·27	0·34	0·38	0.25

Like measles and scarlet fever, whooping cough, although endemic in all large towns, recurs in epidemics. In the two decennia 1861–70–80, there was one such epidemic year in 1866 and a second in 1878. The mortality from whooping cough is highest in the first year of life ; it then diminishes like that of measles, but more rapidly, becoming quite insignificant by the tenth year. It is more fatal in winter, and in towns, and among the poor; but of these differences only the seasonal one is very marked.

Whooping cough resembles diphtheria in the fact that, unlike most zymotic diseases, it is most fatal among females. This is shown in the following table:—

Death-Rate of Males and Females per 1,000 Living from several Zymotic Diseases.

Causes of Death.	1871–80.		1886.	
	Males.	Females.	Males.	Females.
All Causes	22·610	20·000	20·340	18·270
Smallpox	0·267	0·207	0·014	0·006
Measles	0·396	0·360	0·449	0·414
Scarlet Fever	0·750	0·683	0·221	0·209
Diphtheria	0·117	0·125	0·141	0·152
Whooping Cough	0·474	0·547	0·435	0·492
Fever { Typhus Fever	0·494	0·477	0·010	0·007
Fever { Enteric Fever			0·197	0·167
Fever { Continued Fever			0·021	0·023
Diarrhœal Diseases	1·008	0·867	0·975	0·843

Fever.—Under this head are included typhus fever, enteric or typhoid fever, and simple and ill-defined forms of continued fever. These have only been differentiated within the last forty years, and for the earlier years of civil registration it is therefore necessary to consider them together. In the decennium 1871–80, the death-rate from "fever" fell from an annual average of 885 per million to 484—a decline of 45 per cent.—a result which is especially satisfactory, as there are no diseases which are more amenable to sanitary improvements. The following table illustrates the same facts in greater detail:—

England.—Deaths and Death-Rates from Fever (Typhus, Enteric or Typhoid, Simple and Ill-defined), 1850–84.

Year.	Number of Deaths from Fever.	Deaths to 1,000,000 Persons living.	Proportional Number to 1,000 Deaths. Total.
1850	15,374	865	43
1851	17,930	997	46
1852	18,641	1,025	47
1853	18,554	1,008	45
1854	18,893	1,015	44
1855	16,470	875	39
1856	16,182	850	42
1857	19,016	988	46
1858	17,883	918	40
1859	15,877	806	36
1860	13,012	654	31
1861	15,440	767	36
1862	18,721	919	43
1863	18,017	874	38
1864	20,106	963	41
1865	23,034	1,089	47
1866	21,104	986	43
1867	16,862	778	36
1868	19,701	898	41
1869	18,390	828	37
1870	17,910	796	35
1871	15,790	693	31
1872	14,020	607	29
1873	13,553	579	28
1874	13,735	579	26
1875	13,063	543	24
1876	10,746	441	21
1877	9,987	404	20
1878	10,417	416	19
1879	7,933	313	15
1880	8,794	342	17
1881	7,240	278	15
1882	7,992	303	15
1883	7,918	296	15
1884	7,476	276	14
1885	5,745	209	11
1886	5,911	213	11
1887	5,873	207	10

The following table, from the 47th Annual Report of the Registrar-General (1884) shows the decline from fever at different age-groups.

Death-Rate per Million from "Fever" at Different Age-Periods.

Age Periods.	Deaths per Million Living.		Decline per cent. since 1875.
	1875.	1885.	
0–	741	224	70
5–	573	258	55
10–	458	270	41
15–	573	377	34
25–	459	313	32
35–	459	254	45
45–	448	209	53
55–	543	222	59
65–	638	211	67
75–	564	171	70
All Ages	543	276	49

The inequality of the decline of the fever-rate at different ages is probably owing to greater accuracy in diagnosis in regard to the very young and old, who were formerly said to die from "fever," without any further definition of disease, but who are probably now grouped more accurately under other headings. But even after ample allowance for this, there has still been an enormous reduction of fever at all ages. Nor can the reduction of mortality be ascribed to the prevalence of a milder type of disease. If the same test is applied as in the case of scarlet fever; viz., the proportion of cases to deaths in the metropolitan fever hospitals, the case mortality was found to be 180 deaths per 1,000 cases, both in 1875–80 and in 1881–85. The decline in mortality from fever must therefore be due to its diminished prevalence.

Sickness-Rate per 1,000 *of Population from Typhus and Enteric Fever in* 41 *Notification Towns* (Tatham).

	1883.	1884.	1885.	1886.	1887.
Typhus Fever	0·14	0·10	0·11	0·09	0·07
Enteric Fever	1·21	1·55	1·34	1·40	1·29

The mortality from typhus and enteric fever separately for successive years, is given in the table on page 172.

Diarrhœa.—The mortality from diarrhœa in different districts and years is shown in the following table :—

Death-Rate per 1,000 from Diarrhœa in Different Populations.

	1882.	1883.	1884.	1885.	1886.	1887.
England and Wales	0·65	0·60	0·97	0·49	0·88	0·69
London	0·55	0·67	0·97	0·66	0·95	0·90
28 Great Towns . .	0·86	0·77	1·21	0·69	1·16	0·97
50 Other Towns . .	0·78	0·67	1·09	0·47	0·98	0·74
Rural Districts . .	0·48	0·43	0·72	0·34	0·63	0·50

The rates for diarrhœa in England and Wales given above are lower than those given on page 172, for diarrhœal diseases in the corresponding periods, owing to the fact that in the above table deaths returned as cholera have been included with diarrhœa and dysentery. True dysentery was last prevalent as an endemic disease in 1840–47. It may be regarded as practically extinct in this country, except such cases as are imported from tropical and sub-tropical climates. Spite of this, dysentery is frequently seen in death-returns as a cause of death. Such cases are combined in the Registrar-General's returns with the deaths from diarrhœa.

In the decennium 1871–80, the deaths from diarrhœal diseases fell from an annual rate of 1076 to 935 per million, showing an annual gain of 141 lives per million persons living. Diarrhœa is well known to be favoured by hot summers, the mortality from it in London always becoming high when the mean weekly temperature rises to about 63° Fahr.

Now, in the ten years 1861–70 there were, during the three summer months of all these years together, 317 days in which the mean temperature at Greenwich was above 63°, and in the following decennium there were 325 such days; or, adding together all the excess of temperature over 63°, they were in the first decennium 1153°, and in the second 1178°. Thus the two decennia were roughly on an equality as regards temperature, and the reduction in diarrhœal mortality may be fairly ascribed to greater cleanliness and general sanitary improvement (Ogle).

The lowest diarrhœal death-rate, with one exception, recorded within the last 25 years, was in 1885, when it was 487 to a million living, the single exception being 1879, when the rate was 452 per million. In 1879 the mean temperature of the summer months was exceptionally low, especially in August and September, though not quite so low as in 1885. In the 25 years 1861–85 the mean summer temperature was below the 100 years' average in eight years, and the mean of the annual diarrhœa rates in these eight years was 659 per million living, while the mean of the rates in the remaining 17 years was 992 per million.

The connection between a high mean temperature of the air and extent of prevalence of summer diarrhœa is apparently not a direct causal one. In all probability it is rather the putrefactive changes in connection with milk, water, dustbins, etc., which cause the disease.

A deficient rainfall commonly occurs in the years in which diarrhœa is above the average, going along with the excessive temperature of the air.

Diarrhœa Mortality, Mean Temperature and Rainfall in Successive Years in England and Wales. (Meteorological Observations at Greenwich.)

Year.	Death-Rate from Diarrhœa per Million Persons.	Mean Temp. of Air in 3rd Quarter of Year.	Departure from Average of 38 Years.	Annual Fall of Rain in Inches.	Departure from Average of 38 Years.
1880	1171	61·4	+ 1·0	29·8	+ 5·3
1881	558	60·0	− 0·4	25·2	+ 0·7
1882	651	58·1	− 2·3	25·2	+ 0·7
1883	595	59·5	− 0·9	21·9	− 2·6
1884	971	52·7	+ 2·3	18·1	− 6·4
1885	487	59·1	− 1·3	24·0	− 0·5
1886	888	61·2	+ 0·8	24·2	− 0·3
1887	690	61·0	+ 0·8	19·9	− 5·4

The connection between the temperature of the air and the prevalence of diarrhœa is shown in the following diagram :—

DIAGRAM SHOWING WEEKLY MORTALITY FROM DIARRHŒA IN LONDON DURING 1887, COMPARED WITH THE WEEKLY FLUCTUATIONS OF MEAN TEMPERATURE.

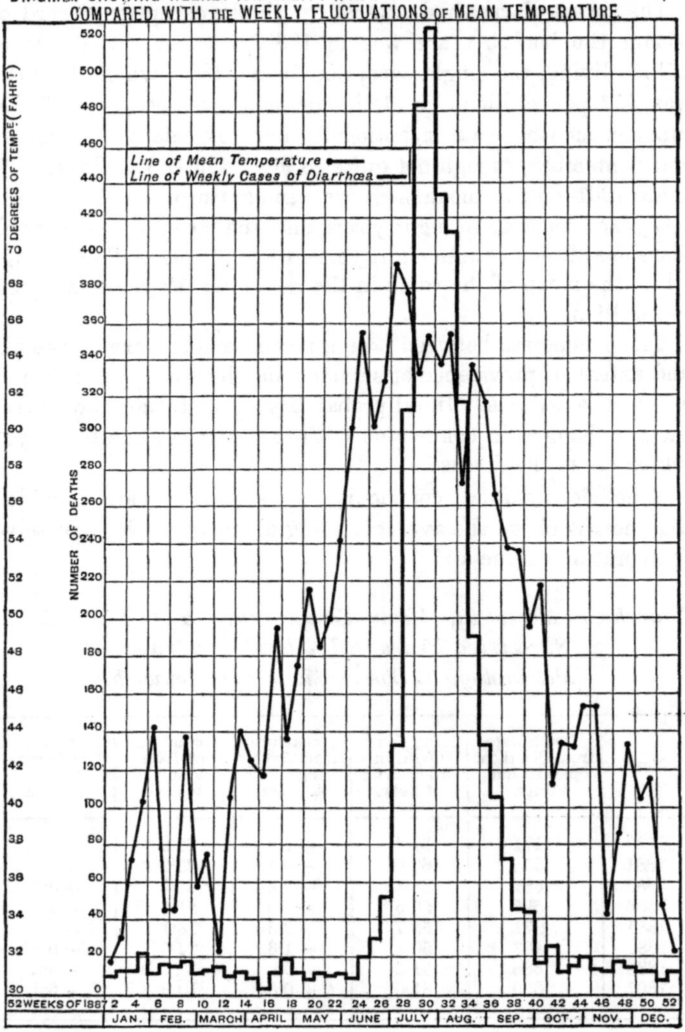

That the connection between deficient rainfall and occurrence of diarrhœa is not constant, is shown by the experience of 1880 in the preceding table. It should be noted, however, that in 1880 there was a deficient rainfall in the two first quarters of the year, and that the greater part of the total excess for the year was in the fourth quarter.

With the exception of 1868, in which it was 1,388, the death-rate from diarrhœa in 1880 was the highest on record. The summer of 1868 was one of extraordinary heat, and the temperature of the summer of 1880 was considerably above the average.

Death-Rate per Million of the Population from Diarrhœa in the 28 great Towns.

	1887.	Ten Years 1877–86.		1887.	Ten Years 1877–86.
Halifax	270	430	Plymouth . . .	1050	710
Huddersfield . .	400	490	Liverpool . . .	1060	1200
Bristol	520	600	Blackburn . . .	1060	1310
Oldham	630	750	Hull	1130	1430
Derby	680	610	Portsmouth . .	1130	900
Newcastle . . .	720	970	Leeds	1150	1270
Birkenhead . .	770	690	Nottingham . .	1200	1090
Norwich . . .	790	1180	Manchester . .	1260	1110
London	900	780	Birmingham . .	1280	1270
Brighton . . .	900	730	Wolverhampton .	1310	1110
Bradford . . .	900	840	Bolton	1390	1400
Cardiff	930	1080	Salford	1490	1520
Sunderland. . .	940	1090	Leicester . . .	1710	1830
Sheffield . .	940	1170	Blackburn . . .	2270	2390

Diarrhœa, as a fatal disease, is pre-eminently an infantile disease, and is one of the chief causes of the excessive infantile mortality in large towns. Of the 29,519 deaths in 1880 from diarrhœa, 18,440, or 62·5 per cent. were of infants in their first year, and 25,998 or 88·1 per cent. of children under five years of age. Of the infants that died of diarrhœa in their first year, 29·5 per cent. were under three months, 31·5 per cent. over three and under six months, while 39 per cent.

were older than this. As there are more infants living under three months than over three and under six months, it appears that diarrhœa is not so destructive of infants in the first as in the second three months of life, which may with probability be ascribed to the greater prevalence of "feeding by hand" after this period of life.

Diarrhœa prevails to a very varying extent in the 28 great towns, as evidenced by the preceding table, in which the towns are arranged in the order of their death-rates per million from diarrhœa.

Such variations are partly due to the varying presence of insanitary conditions, especially those connected with pollution of the soil and the atmosphere with excremental matter; but social reasons also have undoubtedly a great influence, as the occupation of the mothers, the varying amount of feeding by hand, etc. The prevalence of diarrhœa is a matter of great importance, and ought to receive further elaborate and combined investigation by skilled observers.

CHAPTER XII.

SMALLPOX AND VACCINATION.

Smallpox Mortality at Different Periods.—Smallpox Mortality at Different Ages.—Change in the Age-Incidence of Smallpox.—Effect of Vaccination on its Age-Incidence.—Effect of Vaccination on Severity of Smallpox.—Effect of Varying Number of Cicatrices.—Efficient and Inefficient Vaccination.—Why Smallpox not Extirpated.—Proportion of Population Unvaccinated.

PROBABLY no department of vital statistics is so important as that which deals with smallpox and vaccination. As certainly, in no department of medicine has so large an appeal to figures been made, and in none have the deductions from figures been so contradictory.

During 1886 the deaths in England and Wales ascribed to **Smallpox** numbered 275, a number far lower in proportion to the population than in any previous year. There were, however, also 93 deaths ascribed to chickenpox, which probably nearly all of them were in reality smallpox. Even including all these, the death-rate from smallpox would only amount to 13·2 per million living. In the year 1880, the rate per million was 25, the rate in London being 125 per million.

The deaths from smallpox are separated by the Registrar-General into—

Vaccinated.
Unvaccinated.
No Statement.

In 1886, out of 275 deaths from smallpox 25 were registered as vaccinated, 43 as unvaccinated, and concerning 207 there was no statement. In London so large a proportion of the deaths from smallpox occur in hospitals that information can be obtained as to vaccination in about two-thirds of the total deaths.

It will be impossible in this chapter to give more than the chief figures on the subject of smallpox. The reader should refer for fuller details to the Registrar-General's 43rd Annual Report (1880), from which most of the following tables are abstracted; to Dr. Buchanan's Supplement to the 15th Annual Report of the Local Government Board; and for a discussion of the more controversial portions of the subject to Dr. McVail's "Vaccination Vindicated."

In 1880, out of 648 fatal cases of smallpox, in 245 no information was furnished as to vaccination or non-vaccination of the deceased. Of the remaining 403, 282 were certified to have been unvaccinated, and 121 vaccinated. Thus of every hundred fatal cases, concerning which information was available, 70 were unvaccinated, and only 30 vaccinated. Assuming, what is probable, that vaccinated persons in this country are 19 times as numerous as unvaccinated, it follows that the same number of persons who among the vaccinated furnished one death from smallpox, among the unvaccinated furnished 44 deaths. Even assuming that every one of the 245 doubtful cases was really a vaccinated case, the proportion between the two is still as one to fifteen.

Death-Rate per Million Persons in London from all Causes and from Smallpox.

Years.	Average Annual Deaths per Million from All Causes.	Average Annual Deaths per Million from Smallpox.
1660–79	80,000	4,170
1728–57	52,000	4,260
1771–80	50,000	5,020
1801–10	29,200	2,040
1831–35	32,000	830
1838–53	24,900	513
1854–71	24,200	388
1872–82	22,100	262
1883	20,500	136
1884	20,400	1,236
1885	19,800	1,419
1886	19,900	24
1887	19,600	9

Smallpox Mortality at Different Periods.—The preceding table shows the death-rate in London from smallpox for successive periods. The figures given for the years previous to the introduction of the Registration Act were estimated by Dr. Farr.

In the following table the mortality of London from smallpox is compared with that of the provinces.

Deaths from Smallpox per Million of the Population.

Years.	1838–42.	1847–49.	1850–54.	1855–59.	1860–64.	1865–69.	1870–74.	1875–79.	1880–84.
London . . .	755	460	300	237	281	276	654	292	244
Provinces . .	547	274	271	192	175	221	389	48	34

The difference between the metropolitan and provincial mortality in successive periods is brought out more strikingly in the diagram on page 194, reduced from Dr. Buchanan's report to the Local Government Board for 1885.

It will be seen that the decrease in smallpox mortality has been much greater in the provinces than in London. The difference does not appear to be due to any lessened practice or power of vaccination in London as compared with the provinces. This is evidenced by the fact that in London, as in the rest of the country, there is the same greater diminution of deaths from smallpox among children than among adults. The presence of several large smallpox hospitals in London, which have been proved to be foci of infection, may not improbably be an important factor in the greater smallpox mortality in London.

Mortality from Smallpox at Different Ages.—Were the figures already given to form the only basis of comparison for different periods, an insufficient estimate of the diminution in smallpox mortality would be made. It is important, in order to see the full effects of vaccination, that the death-rates from smallpox should be given at successive periods of life. Unfortunately the causes of death were not abstracted in combination with ages until 1847. Since that time vaccination has been in use, and there has been some provision for its

Comparison of London with the Provinces (Buchanan).

Diagram showing mean Annual Smallpox Rates, per million population at all ages, during successive periods since the commencement of Registration. The share of Smallpox Mortality borne by children under five, in each period, is shown in black.

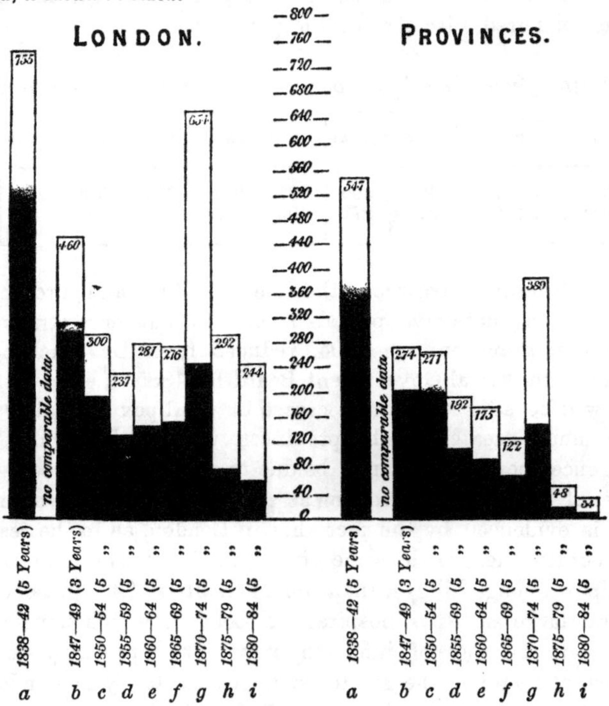

gratuitous performance. We cannot, therefore, compare the smallpox mortality at different age-periods before and after the introduction of vaccination. It is possible, however, to compare periods in which vaccination has been practised to a varying extent. The period from 1847–80 can be divided into three sub-periods:—

1. From 1847–53 inclusive, in which gratuitous vaccination was provided, but recourse to it was purely optional.

2. From 1854–71, in which vaccination was obligatory, but there were no effectual means to enforce the obligation thus instituted.

3. From 1871 onwards, in which vaccination was rigidly enforced, Boards of Guardians being obliged to appoint public vaccination officers in each district.

Mean Annual Deaths from Smallpox at Successive Life-Periods, per Million Living at each such Life-Period.

Sub-Period.	Age						
	All Ages	0–	5–	10–	15–	25–	45 and upwards.
1. Vaccination optional (1847–53)	305	1,617	337	94	109	66	22
2. Vaccination obligatory, but not efficiently enforced (1854–71) .	223	817	243	88	163	131	52
3. Vaccination obligatory, and more efficiently enforced by vaccination officers (1872–80)	156	323	186	98	173	141	58
Entire period of obligatory vaccination (1854–80)	198	633	222	92	167	135	55

It will be evident from the preceding table, that with the gradual extension of vaccination there has been a gradual and notable decline in the death-rate from smallpox at all ages combined, but that this decline is exclusively among children under ten years of age, and indeed chiefly under five years, in which group of ages the mortality fell 80 per cent. in the interval between the first and third period. After the tenth year the mortality has increased, very slightly, from ten to fifteen, very greatly beyond this age; the increase being the greater the more advanced the age. Thus comparing the third with the first period, the rate from fifteen to twenty-five, rose 59 per cent.; from twenty-five to forty-five, rose 114 per cent.; after forty-five, rose 164 per cent.

If, instead of grouping the periods as in the preceding table, a decennial grouping is adopted, the statements as to the change in the age-incidence of smallpox hold good.

Mean Annual Deaths from Smallpox, at Successive Life Periods, per Million Living at each such Life-Period.

	All Ages.	0–	5–	10–	15–	20–	25–	35–	45–	55–	65–	75 and upwards.
1851–60	221	1,034	257	73	93	130	92	53	38	24	18	14
1861–70	163	654	145	56	86	136	102	73	49	36	26	22
1871–80	236	527	284	137	197	300	239	168	111	71	46	35

These changes in the age incidence of smallpox are so great as entirely to preclude any possibility of referring them to errors of registration or fluctuations due to chance. The most natural and probable explanation of them is that vaccination confers an immunity from smallpox in the earlier years of life, which, however, is less complete and permanent than the immunity conferred by an attack of smallpox, thus explaining the increased death-rate from smallpox at the higher ages.

We shall subsequently bring forward evidence confirmatory of the statement that it is vaccination which produces this alteration in the age-incidence of smallpox. In the meantime we must consider the hypothesis which maintains that the decline in smallpox mortality is due, not to vaccination, but to general improvement in the sanitary condition of this country. To begin with, no scrap of evidence is forthcoming, which shows any connection between bad drainage and smallpox. In this respect it is like measles and whooping cough, which remain as prevalent as formerly, spite of the immense strides which have been made in sanitary improvements. Is there any decrease in the case of the other zymotic diseases which is in any measure proportionate to that of smallpox?

The table on page 172 shows that in some of the zymotic diseases there is no decrease, and the only one in which there has been a very striking decrease comparable to that of smallpox is "fever."

If sanitary improvements are the cause of the reduced smallpox mortality, we cannot expect that their effect will be confined to smallpox. There ought to be a similar reduction in the general death-rate *as to distribution as well as amount.* In order to test this, the following table from the Registrar-General's 43rd Report is given. In it the rates of the first sub-period (of optional vaccination, 1847–53) are compared with the rates of the third sub-period (of compulsory vaccination, 1872–80). "Each death-rate in the first sub-period is taken as 100, and the figures in the table give the death-rates in the third sub-period as compared with that 100; in the first line for smallpox, and in the other line for all other diseases together, excepting smallpox."

Death-Rates in 1872–80, *compared with those in* 1847-53, *the latter taken as* 100.

	All Ages.	0–	5–	10–	15–	25–	45–
Smallpox . . .	51	20	55	104	159	214	264
All other Causes	93	94	70	67	71	88	97

At each age-period after ten years the changes in the rates are in opposite directions; while under ten, although in the same direction, they are utterly disproportionate to each other. Taking the deaths at all ages, the death-rate from smallpox fell 49 per cent., while that from other causes fell 7 per cent., so that only one-seventh of the reduction in smallpox mortality could on this supposition be ascribed to improved sanitation.

The correspondence required by the hypothesis plainly does not exist, and the hypothesis itself must therefore fall to the ground. But if the alternative supposition that the great fall in smallpox mortality was due to vaccination is correct, why has the mortality from smallpox among those beyond fifteen years of age actually increased? To begin with, the protection afforded by vaccination is *less perfect* than that afforded by a previous attack of smallpox; and in the next place it is *less permanent.* Its protective influence steadily diminishes, while that of an attack of smallpox appears to remain unaltered. Starting with these facts, the **change in the age-incidence of smallpox** is explained as follows:—

Before the introduction of vaccination but few persons escaped having smallpox at some period of their lives, and the great majority had it when young. Of these a large proportion died, making the smallpox mortality for the early age-periods high; but those who survived, forming a large proportion of the population at the later age-periods, and being permanently protected by an attack of smallpox, made the smallpox death-rate of the later ages a low one. With vaccination the susceptibility of young and old was altered, and in large measure inverted, with a corresponding effect on the smallpox mortality at different ages. The death-rate from smallpox under five fell 80 per cent. between the first and third sub-periods; from five to ten, only 45 per cent. The greater decrease in the first age-period is largely due to the fact that vaccination is now compulsory before the end of the third month of life, formerly not until a year old.

Death-Rate under Five Years of age from Smallpox per Million Children Living under Five, from 1847–1886.

Year.		Death-Rate per Million Living.		Year.		Death-Rate per Million Living.	
		At all Ages.	Under 5.			At all Ages.	Under 5.
1. Vaccination optional . .	1847	430	1,380	2. Vaccination obligatory, but not efficiently enforced . .	1867	440	468
	1848	720	2,097		1868	190	416
	1849	230	1,364		1869	90	297
	1850	210	1,401		1870	300	409
	1851	450	2,067		1871	2,420	2,521
	1852	480	2,124	3. Vaccination obligatory and enforced	1872	540	1,843
	1853	90	893		1873	30	185
2. Vaccination obligatory, but not efficiently enforced . .	1854	280	675		1874	20	169
	1855	410	531		1875	10	83
	1856	200	514		1876	210	185
	1857	60	911		1877	710	316
	1858	90	1,379		1878	390	139
	1859	420	853		1879	120	38
	1860	320	578		1880	120	49
	1861	80	267		1881	620	209
	1862	130	339		1882	110	77
	1863	690	1,176		1883	30	62
	1864	190	1,525		1884	220	139
	1865	210	1,144		1885	220	187
	1866	460	575		1886	10	—

The preceding table shows the change in the relative mortality from smallpox mortality under five years of age, as compared with the entire mortality from this disease during the three sub-periods previously named.

The **effect of vaccination on the age-incidence of smallpox** mortality is shown more strikingly by the following table, based on the records of the seven years (1872–74 and 1877–80), in which alone vaccinated and unvaccinated deaths were abstracted separately:—

Proportion of Deaths under and over Fifteen Years of Age, per 1,000 Deaths from Smallpox in Vaccinated and Unvaccinated Persons respectively.

Age.	Unvaccinated.	Vaccinated.
Under 15	672	334
Over 15	328	666
	1,000	1,000

It is for those who maintain that vaccination is utterly without influence on smallpox to explain how the figures in the preceding table for vaccinated and unvaccinated came to be almost exactly inverted, if their theory is correct.

Percentage of Total Smallpox Mortality borne by Children under Five Years old.

Period.		Percentage of Deaths from Smallpox under 5 to Total Smallpox Deaths in	
		Metropolis.	Provinces.
Vaccination optional .	2 years, 1843–4 . . .	68	?
	5 ,, 1845–9 . . .	68	(yr.1847) 74
	5 ,, 1850–54 . .	65	?
Vaccination obligatory, 1854–71 .	5 ,, 1855–9 . . .	56	57
	5 ,, 1860–4 . . .	53	56
	5 ,, 1865–9 . . .	56	53
Vaccination enforced from 1871.	5 ,, 1870–4 . . .	38	30
	5 ,, 1875–9 . . .	28	29

The preceding figures from Dr. Buchanan's evidence in the "Report of the Hospitals Commission of 1882," present allied facts as to the change of age-incidence of smallpox mortality since the introduction of vaccination, the mean annual mortality from smallpox under 5 being expressed as a percentage of the total smallpox mortality, instead of as a rate per million persons, as in the table on page 198:—

Effect of Vaccination on Severity of Smallpox.—It has been already stated that vaccination does not afford such a complete protection against smallpox as does a previous attack of smallpox. But when a vaccinated person has smallpox, it is usually of a modified and much milder character.

The following table, compiled by Dr. McVail, illustrates this point by the results of hospital experience on a large scale:—

Authority or Hospital.	Total Number of Cases.	Total Mortality per Cent.	Unvaccinated, including those who had Smallpox.		Alleged to be Vaccinated, with or without evidence of Cicatrix.	
			Total.	Mortality per Cent.	Total.	Mortality per Cent.
Mr. Marson (1836-51)	5,795	21·9	2,701	37·2	3,094	8·7
London Smallpox Hospitals (1870-2)	14,808	18·7	3,634	44·8	11,174	10·1
London Smallpox Hospitals (1876-80)	15,171	17·6	3,759	44·4	11,412	8·8
Homerton Hospital (Feb. 1st, 1871, till Dec. 31st, 1877) . .	5,479	19·4	1,243	46·1	4,236	11·5
Deptford Hospital (1881) . . .	3,185	17·3	531	47·4	2,654	11·3
Fulham ,, (1881) . . .	1,752	14·2	210	44·2	1,542	10·1
Dublin ,, (1876-80) . .	2,404	21·7	448	64·2	1,956	12·0

It will be seen that the mortality of the unvaccinated ranges from 37·2 to 64·2 per cent., and of the vaccinated from 8·7 to 12 per cent. Every case was entered as vaccinated, even though there was no mark at all, or a very indifferent one, if vaccination was alleged to have occurred; with the single exception of Dublin, where all cases without cicatrix were entered as unvaccinated.

The following table shows, even more markedly, the effects

of vaccination, and differentiates between the cases in which vaccination marks were good, or imperfect, or not evident. It is a digest of 10,403 cases of smallpox treated by Dr. Gayton in the metropolitan smallpox hospitals:—

Ages.	Vaccinated. Good Marks.			Vaccinated. Imperfect Marks.			"Vaccinated," but no evidence of Vaccination.			Not Vaccinated.		
Years.	Cases.	Deaths.	Per Cent.	Cases.	Deaths.	Per Cent.	Cases.	Deaths.	Per Cent.	Cases.	Deaths.	Per Cent.
0–2	4	0	0	82	8	9	22	9	41	276	181	66
2–5	57	0	0	150	18	12	96	38	40	401	202	50
5–10	206	2	1	582	27	5	207	40	19	510	180	35
10–15	439	5	1	939	32	3	214	42	20	317	74	23
15–20	606	12	2	1,037	66	2	205	39	19	204	86	42
20–25	389	11	3	843	100	13	167	56	34	174	83	48
25–30	189	12	6	529	80	15	116	35	30	105	56	53
30–40	147	14	10	526	78	15	137	49	36	103	42	41
40–50	29	4	14	136	33	18	85	24	28	49	21	43
50+	19	2	11	30	18	22½	46	20	43	30	13	43
All Ages	2,085	62	3	4,854	455	9	1,295	352	27	2,169	938	43

There appears to be a definite connection between the *number of good vaccination cicatrices* and the degree of protection from severe smallpox. This is shown in the preceding table, and even more strikingly in the following table from Mr. Marson's well-known figures, which give "the result of his observations, made during twenty-five years, in nearly 6,000 cases of post-vaccinal smallpox" in the London Smallpox Hospital.

Cases of Smallpox, Classified according to the Vaccination Marks.	Number of Deaths per Cent. in each Class respectively.
Unvaccinated	35½
(1) Stated to have been vaccinated, but having *no* cicatrix	21¾
(2) Having *one* vaccine cicatrix	7½
(3) Having *two* vaccine cicatrices	4⅛
(4) Having *three* vaccine cicatrices	1¾
(5) Having *four or more* vaccine cicatrices	¾

As to Class (2), it is stated that where the one cicatrix was well marked the death-rate was $4\frac{1}{4}$, but where badly marked it was 12 per cent.; and in Class (3) the corresponding figures were $2\frac{3}{4}$ and $7\frac{1}{4}$.

During 1881, 125 children under 10 years of age, died in the London smallpox hospitals from smallpox, who were said to have been vaccinated. A personal investigation of each case was made by Dr. Stevens, with the result that the number was reduced to 117 by the deduction of those who were found not to have been vaccinated, or unsuccessfully vaccinated. Of these 117, 87 had been vaccinated by private practitioners, and 35 by public vaccinators. Now, in London, about equal numbers are vaccinated by public and private vaccinators; while, as shown by the proportion 87 : 35, a more than double mortality fell on those children under 10, who were vaccinated by private practitioners. The children vaccinated by private practitioners belong to well-to-do families, and probably run less risk of smallpox infection than the poor. The discrepancy between the results becomes thus all the more striking. It must be acknowledged that many medical practitioners only produce one or at the most two vesicles, a form of vaccination which is inefficient, and probably responsible for this relatively high mortality from smallpox.

It is worth while to follow further the 35 deaths from smallpox under 10 years of age of children vaccinated by public vaccinators. Of the 35, it turned out that 12 had not been vaccinated until they had been exposed to smallpox, and when it was too late even to modify its virulence. Of the remaining 23 cases, 2 could not be traced, and, in about equal proportions of the remainder, the children were ill of some other disease before the occurrence of what was registered as smallpox, or only imperfect marks were found on their arms. There was only one case in which, although vaccination was apparently efficient, the child died from smallpox. Such an exceptional event is no more a source of surprise than the exceptional occurrence of death from a second attack of smallpox.

Why is not Smallpox Extirpated?—In answering this question, several points should be raised. (1) In the first place, there are certain cases in which neither vaccination, nor even a previous attack of smallpox, appears to confer immunity against a second attack; just as scarlet fever recurs in exceptional cases. (2) A large proportion of the vaccination in this country is only imperfectly executed. (3) The protection afforded by vaccination becomes gradually exhausted, and re-vaccination is not compulsory except among Government *employés.* (4) There is reason to think that a more virulent type of smallpox now occurs, the less resistant varieties of smallpox having been weeded out by vaccination. (5) About five per cent. of the population have never been vaccinated, and these furnish a soil on which smallpox is kept persistently alive.

Every local vaccination officer has to make a return of vaccinations executed during the year to the Local Government Board, as in the following specimen from the returns of the Wandsworth District for the year 1886.

Vaccination Statistics of Wandsworth District.

Sub-Districts.	Number of Births Returned from 1st January to 31st December, 1886.	Successfully Vaccinated.	Insusceptible of Vaccination.	Had Smallpox.	Dead Unvaccinated.	Postponed by Medical Certificate.	Removed to Districts Vaccination Officer of which has been duly apprised.	Removed to places unknown, or which cannot be reached; and cases not having been found.
East Battersea	2,526	2,015	15	..	262	52	7	174
West Battersea	2,626	2,104	11	..	228	66	2	213
Clapham . .	1,092	871	4	..	104	23	8	73
Putney . . .	353	289	2	..	39	7	5	11
Streatham . .	1,091	871	3	..	98	36	23	56
Wandsworth .	1,260	1,042	5	..	120	21	2	70
Totals . .	8,948	6,192	40	..	851	210	47	597

It will be seen that 597 children, or 6·3 per cent. of the whole number, were absolutely unaccounted for; and of the 47 removed to other districts, of which the vaccination officer had been duly informed, and the 210 postponed by medical certificate, doubtless a considerable portion would entirely escape vaccination.

The figures for the whole country are contained in the following table. The percentage of children "unaccounted for" as regards vaccination does not include those postponed under medical certificate.

Percentage of Children "Unaccounted for," nearly all of whom probably remain Unvaccinated.

Year.	London.	Rest of England.
1872	8·8	4 5
1873	8·7	4 2
1874	8·8	4·1
1875	9·3	3·8
1876	6·5	4 0
1877	7·1	4·1
1878	7·1	4·3
1879	7 8	4 5
1880	7·0	4·5
1881	5·7	4·3
1882	6·6	4·5
Average of 5 years 1873–77 . . .	8 1	4·1
Average of 5 years 1878–82 . . .	6·8	4·4

CHAPTER XIII.

MORTALITY FROM SPECIAL DISEASES.

Puerperal Fever and Childbirth.—Hydrophobia.—Cancer.—Increase and Geographical Distribution of Cancer.—Phthisis.—Relation to Damp Subsoil.—Diabetes.—Dietetic Diseases.—Alcoholism.—Developmental Diseases.—Premature Birth.—Local Diseases.—Violence.—Accident.—Suicide.—Homicide.

PUERPERAL Fever.—This name is expunged from the new edition of the nomenclature of the College of Physicians, the use of the terms Pyœmia, Septicæmia, and Erysipelas respectively being advised, with the prefix "Puerperal" in each case. It is doubtful, however, whether such exact definition is in most cases desirable or even possible. Most cases of puerperal fever are undoubtedly septic in origin; but it would usually be difficult to go farther than this in stating their true pathological character. The advice given in the books of forms of certificates of death should however always be followed: "that whenever childbirth has occurred within one month before death, this fact should be registered in connection with the cause of death." This has been to a large extent neglected in the past by medical practitioners, and during the last few years letters sent out from the Registrar-General's office have resulted in two or three hundred deaths being annually added to puerperal fever, which had been previously certified simply as peritonitis, etc.

Puerperal fever being confined to parturient women, it is preferable to calculate the death-rate from it in terms of the number of births rather than of the number of the entire population, as in the following table:—

Annual Number of Deaths of Mothers to 1,000 *Children Born Alive.*

Number of Deaths.	1851–60.	1861–70.	1871–80.	1881.	1882.	1883.	1884.	1885.	1886.	1887.
Puerperal Fever and Childbirth .	4·8	4·69	4·75	4·8	5 09	5·06	4·79	4·98	4·29	4·69
Puerperal Fever .	1·5	1·54	2·07	2·6	2·9	3·0	2 72	2·71	2 39	2 77
Accidents of Childbirth	3·3	3·15	2·68	2·2	2·2	2·1	2·07	2·27	1·90	1·92

Thus in 1887 to every 1,000 children born alive 4·69 deaths of mothers occurred, or one maternal death to 213 live-born children.

It should be remembered that the number of *child-bearings* is not equivalent to the number of births. The births indicate the children born alive. Some other children are stillborn, and some are multiple at birth. Excluding the still births, the number of child-bearings is obtained by reducing the number of births in about the proportion of 1 to 0·9902.

The mortality from puerperal diseases is highest in the 25–35, and in the 35–45 decennia, as shown in the following table, which is founded on the deaths of 116,911 females occurring between 1840 and 1880. (Registrar-General's 50th Report.)

Annual Mortality per Million Living at Different Age-Groups from Puerperal Fever and Childbirth.

All Ages (Standard Million).	10–	15–	20–	25–	35–	45–	5
317	0·3	158	651	932	908	64	0·2

For explanation of the term *standard million* see page 114. During 1887 puerperal fever caused a death-rate of 2·45 per 1,000 inhabitants, and accidents of childbirth of 1·71 per 1,000. The mortality from these causes varies greatly in different parts of the country. It is especially high in North Wales, and generally higher in mining and industrial than in agricultural districts. The official returns probably greatly understate childbirth mortality, the fact of parturition being often omitted from death certificates, and the secondary cause of death alone stated.

Puerperal mortality is largely preventible. The experience of various lying-in hospitals, since the introduction of antiseptic precautions, is ample proof of this. Thus the General Lying-in Hospital, York Road, London, until 1877, was hardly ever free from puerperal fever; it was then shut up for two years, made thoroughly sanitary, and each patient subsequently treated by antiseptic methods, with the result shown in the following table:—

Date.	Number of Confinements.	Number of Deaths.	Average Mortality per 1,000 Deliveries.
1833–60	5,833	180	30·8
1861–77	3,773	64	17 0
1880–87	2,585	16	6·0

Hydrophobia.—The total number of deaths in England and Wales from this disease during 1887 was 29, as against 26 in 1886, and 60 in 1885. The number in 1885 was higher than in any previous year except 1874, when it was 61, and 1877, when it was 79.

Taking the average of the years 1864–86, Lancashire and Cheshire have the largest number of deaths from hydrophobia in proportion to population, the West Riding and Derbyshire also standing high. The Registrar-General remarks: "If a census could be taken of stray dogs, the cause of this distribution would probably be apparent. In London the destruction of 30,000 stray dogs in the nine months beginning with November, 1885, and the compulsory muzzling of all other dogs in the streets, appear to have been most efficacious; for while in 1885 the deaths from hydrophobia registered in London had risen to the unprecedented number of 26, in 1886 they fell to 10; and of these 10, 6 were registered in the first quarter." During the 40 years 1848–87, 990 deaths were registered in

England and Wales from hydrophobia, 785 of males, and 205 of females. Even the highest annual numbers recorded (61 and 79) only give rates of 2·57 and 3·20 per million of the population. The death-rate from homicide during 1887 was 12 per million; so that the risk of losing one's life by murder is three or four times as great as that of losing it from the bite of a rabid animal.

Cancer.—The registered mortality from cancer (including under this name the various forms of malignant disease) has steadily increased, as shown in the following table:—

Mortality from Cancer in England and Wales per Million Living.

	1851–60.	1861–70.	1871–80.	1881.	1882.	1883.	1884.	1885.	1886.	1887.
Males .	195	244	315	364	364	381	405	411	424	456
Females	434	523	622	668	692	702	707	713	733	748
Persons .	317	387	473	520	532	546	559	566	583	606

Thus the mortality registered from cancer is nearly twice as great as that registered 1851–60. Part at least of this increase is, however, only apparent,—due to the improved diagnosis and more careful statement of causes of death. This is shown (1) by the steady decrease in the number of deaths from tumour, abdominal disease, and other ill-defined forms of disease; and (2) by the fact that the increase of mortality from cancer is much greater among males than among females, as shown in the accompanying table:—

Cancer Rates in 1871–80 *compared with those of* 1851–60.

Age-Periods.	Increase per cent.	
	Males.	Females.
35–	39	35
45–	68	39
55–	72	49
65–	74	50
75–	74	52

This greater increase in the male mortality from cancer is most easily understood on the hypothesis that the rise is in great measure apparent and due to better diagnosis; the cancerous affections of males being internal in a much larger proportion than those of females. Had the increase been altogether real, it is difficult to understand why it should affect males so much more than females. The solution of the question whether cancer is really on the increase, as we are inclined to think it is, would be hastened if the Registrar-General were to attempt a classification of cancers according to the part of the body affected; with which object the medical certificate of death should always give information on this point.

Mean Annual Mortality of Males and Females from Cancer per Million Living at Successive Age-Periods.

Age-Periods.	Males.					Females.				
	1851–60.	1861–70.	1871–80.	1881–84.	1848–80.	1851–60.	1861–70.	1871–80.	1881–84.	1848–80.
0–	21	13	13	19	17	23	13	12	16	17
5–	10	8	7	9	9	9	7	7	6	8
10–	8	8	8	12	8	9	8	8	10	8
15–	16	20	18	17	18	18	17	16	16	17
20–	27	27	28	29	27	30	33	27	34	30
25–	63	61	71	70	64	141	163	175	176	159
35–	174	205	241	270	205	592	673	797	849	685
45–	422	539	709	894	553	1,278	1,538	1,771	1,953	1 530
55–	931	1,208	1,598	2,002	1,244	1,853	2,300	2,770	3,146	2,317
65–	1,504	1,877	2,623	3,305	1,998	2,351	2,810	3,538	4,132	2,907
75-	1,749	2,925	3,035	3,449	2,331	2,341	2,823	3,562	4,135	2,900
All Ages	195	244	315	379	255	434	523	622	692	508

The preceding table shows the increase in mortality from cancer in successive decennia, and the greater increase among males. It will be seen also that there is a much greater mortality of females than of males at all age-periods after the 25th year, the influence of sex being most marked from the 25th to the 55th years of life, and greatest about the middle of this period, when the reproductive organs are gradually ceasing their functional activity. The rates for 1848–80 (50th

Report, Registrar-General) given in the above table, are founded on a total of 84,913 male and 187,734 female deaths during that period, the death-rates for this period being per standard million (page 114).

Influence of Age on Cancer Prevalence.—The liability to cancer increases with age; but as the same may be said with equal truth about the liability to death generally, the question is, Does the liability to death from cancer increase more rapidly than the liability to death of all kinds? The answer is given by the following table from the 47th Annual Report of the Registrar-General, which gives the ratio of deaths from cancer to the total deaths at each age-period.

Ratio of Total Deaths to Deaths from Cancer, 1871–80.

Age-Periods.	Total Deaths to one from Cancer.		
	Persons.	Males.	Females.
20–	255	262	248
25–	71	131	49
35–	24	57	15
45–	14	28	9
55–	14	22	10
65–	21	27	17
75 and upwards	48	56	44

It will be seen that the liability to death from cancer increases much more rapidly than the liability to death generally up to the 45–55 age-period; but that after this age the general mortality increases more rapidly than the mortality from cancer.

The Geographical Distribution of Cancer, as shown by the different county rates, requires considerable correction for varying age and sex-distribution, or erroneous conclusions may be arrived at. In the decennium 1871–80, Durham had the lowest cancer mortality; but this is largely explained by its having in its population an exceptionally large proportion of males and of young persons. A table given by the Registrar-General, and with the necessary corrections for age and sex

Mortality from Phthisis and Diseases of the Respiratory System in England and Wales per Million Living at Successive Age-Groups.

Phthisis.

	All Ages.	0–	5–	10–	15–	20–	25–	35–	45–	55–	65–	75–
1848–80 Males	2,443	1,077	448	628	2,093	3,687	3,941	4,089	3,857	3,317	2,152	752
1848–80 Females	2,413	1,033	503	1,077	3,019	3,809	4,175	3,842	2,830	2,124	1,364	546
1851–60 Persons	2,679	1,305	572	1,025	2,961	4,181	4,317	4,091	3,466	2,840	1,983	808
1861–70 ,,	2,475	968	454	825	2,651	3,928	4,243	4,026	3,340	2,656	1,603	539
1871–80 ,,	2,116	767	358	664	2,038	3,117	3,619	3,745	3,132	2,449	1,476	492

Respiratory Diseases.

	All Ages.	0–	5–	10–	15–	20–	25–	35–	45–	55–	65–	75–
1848–80 Males	3,636	11,790	512	195	315	521	830	1,702	3,475	7,455	15,081	25,955
1848–80 Females	2,957	9,885	519	212	299	376	586	1 123	2,266	5,746	12,984	23,055
1851–60 Persons	3,021	10,400	596	230	338	475	672	1 280	2,565	5,790	12,123	19,687
1861–70 ,,	3,364	11,055	551	209	311	449	730	1,415	2,895	6,696	14,071	24,358
1871–80 ,,	3,760	12,204	557	203	301	445	776	1,622	3,255	7,427	16,080	30,241

(47th Report, 1884), shows London at the head of the list, possibly owing to the resort to London for operation of patients from other districts. Against this explanation of the position of London may be mentioned the fact that the counties around the metropolis have a high cancer rate. Mining and industrial counties are, as a rule, low on the list, contrasting favourably with most of the agricultural counties. Eastern counties again have usually a higher cancer mortality than the western, though this rule is not without exceptions. There is a very wide difference between London and Wales; but the Welsh cancer mortality may be low owing to the large number of deaths registered without specification of cause. And, speaking generally, the Registrar-General sums up the result of his inquiry thus: "It must be confessed that, notwithstanding all the labour that has been expended in duly correcting the cancer mortality in the several counties for differences of age and sex distribution of their respective populations, no certain conclusions can be drawn from the results."

Phthisis.—The death-rates for phthisis for the period 1848–80 (p. 211), are calculated on the basis of the 827,394 male and 874,633 female deaths from phthisis which occurred during this period; and the rates for respiratory diseases on 1,226,324 male and 1,067,493 female deaths from respiratory diseases which occurred during the same period. Being calculated on such an extensive basis, they are of great value.

The preceding table shows an annual gain of 563 lives per million of the population, when the 1871–80 period is contrasted with the 1851–60 period. This is, however, more than counterbalanced by the loss of 739 additional lives per million from respiratory diseases. During 1887 the deaths from phthisis were only 1,591 per million, the lowest mortality yet recorded from this disease; while the mortality from respiratory diseases in this year was 3,572 per million. The increase in respiratory diseases, coincident with the diminution in phthisis, renders it probable that, owing to more accurate statement of causes of death, there has been considerable transference from one to the other. The term phthisis is now not so loosely used as formerly, when any chronic chest affection received this name. But that this is by no means a complete explanation of the decrease in phthisis, is evidenced by the fact that while the mortality from phthisis has decreased at all age-groups, the mortality from respiratory diseases has only increased under 5 and over 35 years of age. And it will be noticed also that the mortality from phthisis chiefly takes place between the ages of 15–55 years, while that from respiratory diseases is very low during these years, and greatest at the extremes of life.

Mortality from Phthisis, Other Tubercular Diseases, and Respiratory Diseases per Million Persons Living at all Ages.

	1851–60.	1861–70.	1871–80.	1881.	1882.	1883.	1884.	1885.	1886.	1887.
Phthisis . .	2,679	2,475	2,116	1,825	1,844	1,870	1,812	1,752	1,718	1,591
Other Tubercular Diseases.	804	784	762	705	729	707	738	654	726	658
Diseases of Respiratory System.	3,021	3,364	3,760	3,427	3,555	3,656	3,317	3,699	3,594	3,572

Other forms of tubercular and scrofulous diseases have not diminished to the same extent as phthisis; and if hydrocephalus had been stated separately in the preceding table, there would have been no decrease in the remaining tubercular diseases during the period 1851–80.

The table of *age*-distribution of phthisis (p. 211) shows that it reaches its maximum mortality between the ages 25-45. There is, as pointed out by the Registrar-General (50th Report) a remarkable difference in *sex*-mortality; the female mortality from 5–35 being in considerable excess of the male, after which time the male mortality is the higher.

It was long ago shown by Dr. Greenhow that in proportion as the male and female population are severally attracted to *indoor* branches of industry, other things being equal, their respective death-rates from phthisis are increased. The effect of sanitary measures, involving drying of the subsoil in decreasing the prevalence of phthisis has been already stated (page 129). Some doubt has been thrown on the active part played by a *damp subsoil* in the etiology of phthisis by Dr. Kelly's observations (p. 120).

The amount of fatality due to phthisis is still extremely great. With the exception of diseases of the respiratory system, it carries off more victims than any other disease. All tubercular diseases massed together, caused 11·9 per cent. of the entire mortality in 1887. During the same year phthisis caused 44,935 deaths out of a total of 530,758, or 8·4 per cent. of the total mortality. During the same year respiratory diseases (not including croup) caused 100,892 deaths, or 19 per cent. of the total mortality.

Diabetes.—The death-rate from diabetes mellitus has steadily increased during the last twenty years. In 1887 it was 62 per million, the highest yet recorded. Much of this apparent increase is doubtless due to greater care in diagnosis and in certification; but it is also suggested that there has been a real increase due to the increased mental strain and worry of modern life, a similar explanation being given for the increase of chronic renal disease. The Registrar-General points out, however—what somewhat invalidates this assumption—that the increase under these headings has been fully as great among children under 5 years, as at school ages or in adults.

During the thirty years 1856–85, 25,100 deaths resulted from diabetes mellitus in England and Wales, the average annual death-rate per million living being, for males, 48; for females, 26; which gives a proportion of male to female mortality of 185 : 100. In each sex the death-rate from this disease increases steadily at each age-period until 65–75, when the rate is at its maximum. Except under 5, there is a great excess in the male death-rate, the difference increasing with age. The mean annual mortality from diabetes in England and Wales is 26 per cent. above that of Scotland and 40 per cent. above that of Ireland. Apparently there is a remarkable inverse relation between the amount of diabetes and the amount of rainfall, which agrees with the relative distribution in the three countries (Registrar-General's 48th Report, 1885).

Dietetic Diseases.—These may be classified as deaths from deficiency of diet (scurvy, starvation, want of breast-milk) and deaths from excess of diet, of which the most important is alcoholism. In 1887, 1,442 deaths were ascribed to intemperance and 323 to other dietetic diseases, giving a death-rate of 63 per million living. The deaths returned under this head are, however, not trustworthy; alcoholism causes in reality an enormously greater mortality than is ascribed to it. One of the commonest diseases due to alcoholism is *cirrhosis of the liver*; and as this is the chief cause of mortality under the heading "liver diseases and ascites," the latter may be taken as a fairly correct index of the amount of alcoholic excess in England and Wales.

Annual Death-Rate per Million Persons Living from Diseases of the Liver and Ascites.

Period.	3 years. 1858–60.	5 years. 1861–65.	5 years. 1866–70.	5 years. 1871–75.	5 years. 1876–80.	5 years. 1881–85.	1886.	1887.
Death-Rate per Million	394·0	416·0	417·6	427·8	423·6	370·0	355	332

It will be seen that the mortality from liver diseases has been declining for some years. The inference that the alcoholic habits of the people are improving is borne out by the fact that the Board of Trade returns show a large diminution in the consumption of drink, and the census returns a large falling off in the number of persons engaged in the liquor trade (a decline equal to 17·9 per cent. for equal populations between 1871 and 1881).

Developmental Diseases.—The following table shows that the death-rate from premature birth has steadily increased, being higher in 1887 than in any previous year. This is all the more striking when the low birth-rate of recent years is taken into account. The best way to estimate the number of deaths resulting from premature birth is *in proportion to the total number of births.* Expressed in this way, we find that the proportion of deaths from premature births in 1861–65 was 11·19 to 1,000 births; since which time it has steadily increased, reaching the ratio of 15·89 per 1,000 births in 1887. This progressive increase in deaths from premature birth may be connected with the markedly increased employment of women in industrial occupations. It has been surmised, however, that as the infantile mortality from all causes together has not been increased, part of the increased mortality from premature birth is only apparent, and due to transference from other headings.

Annual Death-Rate per Million Persons Living from

Cause of Death.	1858–60.	1861–65.	1866–70.	1871–75.	1876–80.	1881–85.	1886	1887.
Premature Birth . .	378 7	392 4	406·0	416 8	472·8	472·8	489	499
Atelectasis . .	?	?	?	?	?	23·4	24	25
Congenital Malformation	57·7	61·6	64·8	65·6	84·4	84 0	84	77
Old Age . . .	1,422	1,353	1,276	1,207	1,072	1,009	1,021	954

The above table shows a falling off in the death-rate from *old age*. If this were a real falling off, it would not be an indisputable advantage, as most people would prefer to die of old age. The decline under this head is, however, chiefly due to an improved specification of the causes of which the old die. The mortality "from old age" is always higher in cold seasons, cold being the special enemy of the old, as heat is of the young.

Local Diseases.—Among the many large groups of diseases included under this head, nervous circulatory and urinary diseases show year by year an almost uninterrupted increase. In the years 1881–85 there were 252 more deaths per million from **nervous diseases** than 20 years earlier. Of this excess, 112 deaths were under 5 and 93 over 65, the increase being at the extremes of age. The Registrar-General concludes from this (49th Report) that much of the increase is apparent, and is probably connected with the decrease in the death-rate from convulsions in the 0–5 group and from old age over 65. When, however, the mortality at different age-groups for 1871–80 is compared with the corresponding rates for 1861–70, there is seen to be a considerable increase from 35 onwards, which must be regarded as partly real, and not entirely due to greater care in statement of cause of death.

Much of the increase under the head of **Circulatory Diseases** is probably due to transference from such headings as Debility, Old Age, and the like, which assumption is supported by the fact that the main increase is in the later age-periods. Some of the increase is also possibly due to the institution of letters of inquiry from the General Register Office when "Dropsy" was returned as the cause of death.

In regard to **Urinary Diseases**, we have also to bear in mind the diminution under the heading "Dropsy," though there is possibly a real increase in mortality from urinary diseases. The uncertain amount of allowance for transference of diseases (due to better diagnosis or more careful certification) is a stumbling-block at every step. The weighty remarks of the Registrar-General on this point may be quoted: "to be without trustworthy means of comparison is doubtless an evil, but to ignore the differences and to deal with the records as thoroughly reliable would be still worse, for it is far better to be without statistics at all, than to be misled by false ones."

Violence.—The following table shows the death-rate from the various forms of violence in successive year-periods.

Mean Annual Death-Rate per Million Living from Violence.

	1858–60.	1861–65.	1866–70.	1871–75.	1876–80	1881–85.	1886.	1887.
Accident and Negligence	653·0	639·6	677·8	670·6	630·4	576·6	534	549
Homicide . .	18·0	19·4	19·0	16·6	14·0	12·6	11	12
Suicide. . .	65·3	65·2	66·4	66·0	73·6	73·8	80	80
Execution. .	0·3	0·8	0·4	0·4	1·0	0·4	1	1

In 1887, 18,125 deaths were ascribed to violence, or 642 per million living. The death-rate from violence is much lower among females (only one-third that of males) and higher under

10 years of age. Occupation, however, has a much greater influence on the number of deaths from violence than diverse age and sex-distribution. Mining raises the rate most; next come quarrying and fishing.

Accident caused 15,518 deaths in 1887. The rate per million was 808 for males and only 304 for females. The influence of *age and sex* is shown by the following facts respecting the quinquennium 1878–82. Under one year of age the fatal accidents of boys are 6 per cent. more numerous than those of girls—a difference closely corresponding to the relative number of boys and girls living at that age. In the second year of life the accidents of boys are 30 per cent. more numerous, in the third year 51 per cent., in the fourth year 61 per cent., and in the fifth year 75 per cent. more numerous than the accidents of girls. After this the preponderance of accidents of males becomes greater, the influence of occupation coming into action. The higher male mortality from accident is no explanation of the higher general death-rate of males, the total mortality from violence being too small to affect the general death-rate to any great extent, and the difference from this cause being partly counterbalanced by the mortality of females from childbirth and puerperal fever. During the decennium 1871–80, the mean annual death-rate was, for males, 22·61; for females, 20·00 per 1,000. If there had been no deaths from violence or from childbirth and puerperal fever, these rates would have been 21·49 and 19·32 respectively.

Of the 549 deaths per million persons due to accident in 1889, 238 per million were caused by fractures and contusions, 4 by gunshot wounds, 6 by cuts or stabs, 82 by burns or scalds, 13 by poison, 94 by drowning, 66 by suffocation, and 46 per million otherwise. Mining operations, vehicles, burns, scalds, and explosions and drowning, were the most common causes of accident.

To **suicide** in 1887 were ascribed 2,234 deaths, or 80 per million living: for males, 122; and for females, 39 per million living. Not only has the death-rate from suicide increased, but also the proportion of male to female suicides has increased.

For both sexes the tendency to commit suicide appears to increase up to the age of 65–75 years, diminishing as the natural end of life approaches (45th Report, Registrar-General).

Mean Annual Suicides of Males and Females at Successive Periods of Life, per Million of the Sex Living at each Period, 1871–80.

Period of Life.	Rate per Million Living.		Of Equal Numbers Living, Male Suicides to 100 Female Suicides.
	Males.	Females.	
0–	0·00	0·00	—
10–	3·54	2·80	126
15–	24·74	24·20	102
20–	65·16	32·93	198
25–	104·43	36·71	284
35–	179·69	52·99	339
45–	267·76	78·30	342
55–	405·94	97·80	415
65–	408·12	98·27	415
75–	336·75	86·77	388
85 and upwards	239·48	64·59	371

The two sexes also show marked differences as to the methods they adopt in destroying themselves, women commonly avoiding weapons and adopting poison or drowning in greater proportion than the other sex (45th Report).

Method of Suicide Adopted by Males and by Females, per 1,000 *Suicides of each Sex*, 1871–80.

Method.	Males.	Females.
Hanging, Strangulation	399·3	268·1
Cut, Stab, or other Wound	212·0	147·9
Drowning	165·5	333·3
Poison	78·9	172·2
Gunshot	67·8	2·3
Lying on Rail, or Jumping from Train	23·6	7·6
Jumping from Height	20·5	35·9
Otherwise	31·9	32·7

In regard to poisons, there are wide differences between the sexes, probably owing to the fact that males have freer access to and therefore a wider choice of poisons, and are also better informed on the subject. Out of every 1,000 males who poisoned themselves during 1871–80, 567 used narcotic poisons; while of 1,000 women who poisoned themselves, only 246 had recourse to these. On the other hand, strychnine, or vermin killer, arsenic and phosphorus, carbolic acid and vitriol, spite of the acute sufferings they produce, were used by women in 544 cases out of 1,000, against 246 cases out of 1,000 in which they were used by male suicides.

As regards the local distribution of suicide, the total deaths from this cause in each county are too small to form a trustworthy basis for calculation. It would appear, however, that suicide is much more common in the educated than in the uneducated classes (Registrar-General's 45th Report), as shown in the following table:—

Education and Suicide.

Counties Grouped by Educational Condition.	Mean Annual Suicides per Million Living.
Counties where as many as 27 per cent. were unable to sign Marriage Register	57·5
Counties where less than 27 per cent., but more than 17 per cent., were unable to sign Register	69·2
Counties where less than 17 per cent. were unable to sign Register	80·3

N.B.—The proportions of persons unable to write are the averages of the 10 years 1869–78.

Homicide (including manslaughter and murder) was the registered cause of 352 deaths in 1887, or 12 per million persons, 199 being returned as murder and 153 as manslaughter.

By **execution** 21 deaths occurred during 1887, a larger number than in any year since 1877. In the 24 years, 1863–86, only one criminal was hanged to 15·5 recognised murders, while the proportion was 1 to 9·5 murders in 1887.

CHAPTER XIV.

LIFE TABLES.

Dr. Farr's Biometer.—Data for Life Table.—Method of Construction of Life Table.—Shorter Method of Dr. Farr.—Mr. Noel Humphrey's Method.—History of Life Tables.—Halley.—De Moivre's Hypothesis.—Dr. Price's Northampton Table.—Mr. Milne's Carlisle Table.—Dr. Farr's English Life Tables No. 1 and No. 2.—English Life Table No. 3.—Normal or Life-Table Population.—Healthy Districts Life Table.—Upper-Class Experience Table.—Healthy Males Table.—Clerical Experience Table.—Dr. Ogle's New English Life Table.

LIFE **Tables** afford an accurate means of measuring the probabilities of life and death. They represent "a generation of individuals passing through time," the data on which they are founded being the number and ages of the living, and the number and ages of the dying. Dr. Farr calls the Life Table a *biometer*, and speaks of it as of equal importance, in all inquiries connected with human life or sanitary improvements, with the barometer or thermometer and similar instruments employed in physical research; and as being also the keystone or pivot on which the whole science of life assurance hinges. Even supposing that an insurance society had empirically arrived at an equitable rate of premium for assuring lives, the Mortality or Life Table is still required in order to ascertain the value of such premiums for a prospective term of years, as against the value of the sums assured thereby, so that a statement of assets and liabilities may be periodically prepared. Without such knowledge a division of "profits" would be impossible. In fact the Life Table is absolutely essential for "the solution of all questions depending on the duration of human life."

Addison in his "Vision of Mirza," possibly writing with Halley's graduated Life Table before him, gives the following allegory:—

"The bridge thou seest, said he, is *Human Life*; consider it attentively. Upon a more leisurely survey of it, I found that it consisted of *threescore and ten entire arches*, with several broken arches, which, added to those that were entire, made up the number *about an hundred.* As I was counting the arches, the Genius told me that this bridge consisted at first of a *thousand arches;* but that a great flood swept away the rest, and left the bridge in the ruinous condition I now beheld it. But tell me further, said he, what thou discoverest on it. I see multitudes of people passing over it, said I, and a black cloud hanging on each end of it. As I looked more attentively, I saw several of the passengers dropping through the bridge into the great tide that flowed underneath it: and upon further examination perceived that there were innumerable trap-doors that lay concealed in the bridge which the passengers no sooner trod upon, but they fell through them into the tide, and immediately disappeared. These hidden pit-falls were set very thick at the entrance of the bridge, so that throngs of people no sooner break through the cloud, but many of them fell into them. They grew *thinner towards the middle*, but multiplied and laid closer together towards the end of the arches that were entire. There were, indeed, some persons, but their number was very small, that continued a kind of hobbling march of the broken arches, but fell through one after another, being quite tired and spent with so long a walk."

Without discussing the duration of life in the antediluvian age, we have here a graphic narration of the "hidden pitfalls and trap-doors," and the "broken arches," which beset the course of human life, and the beautiful simplicity of the description forms a useful comment on the diagram at page 236–7.

Description of Life Table.—The essential portions of a Life or Mortality Table are the number and ages of the living and the number and ages of the dying.

1. Suppose that we could observe a million children, all born

at the same moment, and follow them throughout life, entering in a column the number who remain alive at the end of each successive year until all have died. This column is headed by the symbol l_x; where l_x represents the number who reach the precise age x.

In a second column we record the number dying before the completion of each year of life. Thus the number who die before reaching the first anniversary are placed opposite the age 0 in the table, and so on. In this way we obtain the column headed d_x; where d_x represents the number out of l_x persons attaining the precise age x, who die before reaching the age $x+1$. It is evident, therefore, that—

$$d_x = l_x - l_{x+1}$$

i.e., the number dying between the ages x and $x+1$ is equal to the difference between the numbers living at the ages x and $x+1$.

In practice it is not possible to observe a body of children throughout life in the precise manner indicated, so that other methods must be resorted to.

2. It is not necessary to assume, as in the preceding case, that all the persons observed have been born at the same time. If we could trace any 1,000,000 children throughout life, however various might be the dates of their births, a Life Table might be similarly constructed, if the numbers living and dying during each year of life were known.

Our national records do not lend themselves to this method, but Friendly Societies and Life Assurance Offices, as well as Annuity and Pension Institutions, afford the requisite data for observing individual lives and thus constructing a trustworthy Life Table, though seldom in so complete a form as to cover the whole period of life from birth to death.

3. Without tracing the history of individual children through life, we may, by taking a complete census of the population, distributed according to age and sex, obtain data for forming the column l_x. Similarly, from the annual death-returns, we obtain the number dying during each year of life, and thus form

the column d_x; and from these data can estimate the number of deaths *per unit of population* which forms the column headed m_x.*

The method usually adopted in constructing a Life Table is a modification of this. The number of persons dying within a given period and their ages at death are observed, and it is assumed that the mortality for any year of age thus obtained will be applicable to other lives in the Table, as they successively attain the age in question. In the same way the number out of a million persons, living at each age or group of ages is ascertained from a single census or by combining the results of two or more census enumerations. By these means results are obtained which, being wholly based on recent observations, will probably be more correct, as indicating the present conditions affecting the duration of life, than if a million persons were watched from birth to death; for, in the latter case, the conditions which determined the rate of mortality might, before the series was available, have undergone great changes, and for practical purposes the table be almost valueless.

Dr. Farr's English Life Table, No. 3, was based on the registered deaths in England and Wales during the seventeen years 1838–54, and on the two census enumerations of population in 1841 and 1851. Dr. Ogle's Life Table is based on the mean population of the decennium 1871–80, and on the total deaths during the same decennium. A comparative view of these two tables is given on page 238.

Method of Construction of Life Table.—It is evident that the deaths in a population, during any stated year, do not occur simultaneously either at the beginning or the end of the year, but are distributed throughout its course. It is also evident

* The ratio of deaths to mean population, or m_x, has been called by Farr the rate of mortality, and we follow his notation and system; but actuarial writers reserve the name *rate of mortality* for the probability of dying within a year (q_x). The name *central death-rate* has been given by these writers to m_x, because it represents the rate at which people are dying in the *centre* of the year x to $x+1$.

that the deaths registered at any age x will not have occurred at the precise age x, but some will have just attained the age x, whilst others will have been close on $x+1$. Now it is assumed, in the usual method of constructing a Life Table, that the deaths at age x occur at equal intervals throughout the ensuing year, so that data may be extracted from the death-registers strictly analogous to their ultimate form (d_x) in the Life Table.

With regard to the "numbers living," however, it is not so. As we have seen, l_x in the Life Table is the number who, out of a given number born, attain the precise age x. The number l_{10} represents the number surviving to the end of their tenth year out of a given number l_o at birth. But in a population situated as just described, persons will be found whose ages are of various intermediate periods between x and $x+1$, or in the instance taken, between ten and eleven years. If, however, we assume the deaths to be equally distributed throughout the year, the number who attain its middle will be the arithmetical mean of those commencing the year and those completing it. Thus—

$$l_{x+\frac{1}{2}}=\frac{1}{2}\,(l_x+l_{x+1}).$$

The number who attain the middle of the tenth year of life is $l_{10\frac{1}{2}}=\frac{1}{2}\,(l_{10}+l_{11})$. We will denote the *mean population* thus obtained by L_x and the deaths extracted from the registers by D_x.

The assumption of a uniform distribution of deaths introduces an error. If, for instance, the deaths in the eleventh year are more numerous than in the tenth, then the deaths towards the close of the tenth year will be more numerous than in any equal period towards the commencement of the same year. Except perhaps for the first two years of life, this error is, however, infinitesimal in amount, and for practical purposes may be disregarded.

If now we divide the deaths registered at any year of age (D_x) by the mean population found existing at that year of age

(L_x), we shall ascertain the rate at which the population is dying in the centre of that year of age. Thus we have—

$$\frac{D_x}{L_x}=m_x \text{ where } m_x=\text{rate of mortality per unit of population.}$$

We have already stated that the Life Table enables us to measure the probabilities of life and of death; and, conversely, having given these probabilities, we can construct the Life Table. We must first, however, see how these probabilities may be calculated from the rate of mortality (m_x) already obtained.

Now the probability of an event occurring is represented by a fraction whose denominator is the number of possible events, and numerator the number of favourable events. Thus, if there are 8 balls in a bag, of which 3 are black and 5 white, the probability of drawing a white ball is found as follows. The number of possible drawings is 8, inasmuch as any one of the balls may be drawn, but only 5 of these would be favourable. Hence the probability$=\frac{5}{8}$.

The probability of drawing a black ball$=1-\frac{5}{8}=\frac{3}{8}$

Reverting now to the symbols and conditions of the Life Table, let l_x=number of persons living at the beginning of the year $\frac{x+1}{}$, of whom l_{x+1} survive to the end of the year. The probability of any one living to the end of the year is therefore $\frac{l_{x+1}}{l_x}$; and inasmuch as d_x die during the year, the probability of any one dying during the year is $\frac{d_x}{l_x}$.

If we indicate by p_x the probability that a person of the precise age x will survive one full year, and by q_x the probability that the same person will die within one year, then—

$$p_x=\frac{l_{x+1}}{l_x}$$

$$q_x=\frac{d_x}{l_x}$$

$$\left.\begin{array}{l}\text{Thus the probability of}\\ \text{living through one year}\end{array}\right\}=\frac{\text{number of survivors at end of year}}{\text{number living at beginning of year}}$$

$$=\frac{l_{x+1}}{l_x}=\frac{l_x-d_x}{l_x}=p_x$$

$$\text{Now } \frac{l_x-d_x}{l_x}=\frac{(l_x-\frac{1}{2}d_x)-\frac{1}{2}d_x}{(l_x-\frac{1}{2}d_x)+\frac{1}{2}d_x}$$

Now if from the precise number living at age x we deduct one-half of the deaths occurring in the ensuing year, we plainly arrive, on the assumption of a uniform distribution of deaths at the "mean population" of the year.

Hence, $l_x-\frac{1}{2}d_x$, which may also be written $\frac{1}{2}(l_x+l_{x+1})$ $=$the mean population for the year, which is denoted by $l_{x+\frac{1}{2}}$.

$$\text{Therefore } p_x=\frac{l_{x+\frac{1}{2}}-\frac{1}{2}d_x}{l_{x+\frac{1}{2}}+\frac{1}{2}d_x}$$

Dividing each term by $l_{x+\frac{1}{2}}$, we obtain—

$$p_x=\frac{1-\frac{1}{2}\frac{d_x}{l_{x+\frac{1}{2}}}}{1+\frac{1}{2}\frac{d_x}{l_{x+\frac{1}{2}}}}$$

$$\text{But the fraction } \frac{d_x}{l_{x+\frac{1}{2}}}=\frac{\text{number dying at age } x}{\text{mean population at age } x}=m_x$$

i.e., the rate at which people are dying in the middle of the year of age x to $x+1$; and this is the same rate as that previously arrived at by dividing the D_x of the death-registers by the L_x ascertained by enumerating the population. Hence we have—

$$p_x=\frac{1-\frac{1}{2}m_x}{1+\frac{1}{2}m_x}=\frac{2-m_x}{2+m_x}$$

By this formula a very simple relation is found to exist between the probabilities of life and the rate of mortality. Having, from the census returns and the death registers, obtained the ratio m_x for all values of x (*i.e.*, all ages), we can by the above formula find p_x, and thence we can, by continued multiplication, construct the Life Table.

This method may be made clearer by an example. The entry in the m_x column is obtained by dividing the deaths during the year by the mean population. From the entry in this column p_x, or the probability of living one year, is obtained by the formula $p_x=\frac{2-m_x}{2+m_x}$. Thus at birth the probability of a male living one year is, by the English Life Table, $\frac{2-\cdot18326}{2+\cdot18326}=\cdot83212$, and for each year in the series the probability of living one year is obtained in the same way.

The next column (l_x) is obtained by multiplying the number living at the immediately preceding year by p_x. Thus, starting with 511,745 males at birth, the number living at the end of one year is obtained by multiplying the probability of surviving to the end of the first year by this number ($l_1=l_0\times p_1$)

$$511745\times\cdot83212=425358\cdot6.$$

This process is shortened by logarithms as follows:—

$$\text{Log. } 511745=5\cdot7085692$$
$$\text{Log. } \cdot83212=\bar{1}\cdot9201860$$
$$\text{Log. of product of these two}=5\cdot6287552$$
$$\text{Therefore product}=425358\cdot6$$

The next column required in a Life Table is one showing the mean number living in each year of life (technically called P_x). Thus the mean number living in the 21st year$=\frac{l_{20}+l_{21}}{2}$.

The next column in the Table is known as the Q_x column. The number opposite any age in this column is the sum of all the numbers in the P_x column from that age to the end of the Table, *i.e.*, until all the lives become extinct; and it shows, therefore, the aggregate number of years which the persons at each age in the Table will live. Thus—

$$Q_x=l_{x+1}+l_{x+2}+l_{x+3}+\text{etc.}+l_{x+n}$$

where $x+n$=the last age mentioned in the Life Table.

From the column (Q_x), and the l_x column, the mean future lifetime (expectation of life) of any person can be obtained by the formula $\frac{Q_x}{l_x}$.

Thus the total future lifetime of all males at birth= 20,426,138 years, and the number of males in the table=511,745; therefore the expectation of life at birth$=\frac{20426138}{511745}=31{\cdot}91$ years.

Similarly the total future lifetime of all males at 20 years of age=13169656, and the number of males living at this age =333608; therefore the expectation of life at the age of 20 years$=\frac{13169656}{333608}=39{\cdot}48$ years.

Besides representing the total number of years to be passed through by the persons living at a certain age, the column Q_x may be regarded as showing the total population of the community. For instance, if 511,745 births take place annually, this shows us that, eventually, the total male population, existing at any particular moment, will be 20,426,138. Again, if it were required to find what standing army of men aged 20 to 45, could be maintained out of the total male population, we find in the column Q_x that the number

aged 20 and upwards is	13,169,656
and „ 45 „ „	5,774,489
The difference gives the required number=	7,395,167

The column Q_x provides a solution for many similar problems; but it must be borne in mind, that it assumes a stationary population; *i.e.*, a population annually recruited by the same number of births, a condition which never actually occurs in practice.

The following table is an extract from Dr. Farr's English Life Table No. 3, with the addition of two columns, showing respectively p_x and E_x, which have been introduced in order to give a complete view of the results obtainable from a Life Table. Each year of age should be inserted, in order to make it complete, but the reader is referred to Dr. Farr's English Life Tables for the complete data.

Dr. Farr's English Life Tables for Males.

Age (or Past Life-time.) (x)	Annual Mortality per Unit at Age x $=m_x$	Probability of Living One year from each age $=p_x$	Number Born and Living at each age $=l_x$	Mean Population in each year of age $l_{x+\frac{1}{2}}$ $=P_x$	Years which the Males at each age will live $=Q_x$	Mean After lifetime of Males of the age x $E_x=\frac{Q_x}{l_x}$
0	·18326	·83212	511,745	456,820	20,426,138	39·91
5	·01369	·98640	370,358	367,672	18,410,252	49·71
10	·00563	·99438	353,031	352,007	16,608,936	47·01
15	.00519	·99482	344,290	343,415	14,866,429	43·18
20	·00832	·99171	333,608	332,231	13,169,656	39·48
25	·00920	·99084	319,442	317,892	11,536,677	36·12
35	·01105	·98901	288,850	287,229	8,492,601	29·40
45	·01554	·98458	253,708	251,763	5,774,489	22·76
55	·02485	·97644	209,539	206,984	3,447,708	16·45
65	·04698	·95410	150,754	147,315	1,631,508	10·82
75	·10391	·90122	75,777	72,012	491,685	6·49
85	·21966	·80208	16,877	15,151	63,030	3·73
95	·42035	·65265	833	678	1,806	2·17
105	—	—	4	3	5	

The labour involved in constructing a detailed Life Table after the method just described is very great, and the following **shorter method of Dr. Farr**, giving the necessary data for quinquennial periods up to 15, and after that age for decennial periods, is useful in the construction of local Life Tables for comparison with the one for England and Wales.

The probability of living through one year$=\frac{2-m}{2+m}$.

Similarly, the probability of living through a second year$=\frac{2-m}{2+m}$.

The probability of living through the two years is the product of these$=\left(\frac{2-m}{2+m}\right)\left(\frac{2-m}{2+m}\right)$

But the value of m is not the same in these two factors (as the rate of mortality per unit varies from year to year of life). If, however, we take m_1 to represent the mean of these two values of m, each factor will then become—

$$\left(\frac{2-m_1}{2+m_1}\right)\left(\frac{(2-m_1)}{2+m_1}\right)=\left(\frac{2-m_1}{2+m_1}\right)^2$$

which may be taken as a near approximation to the truth. Similarly, for 5 or 10 years, the mean annual death-rate per unit for this group of years is taken; and if the value of this be represented by μ in one case the formula $\left(\frac{2-\mu}{2+\mu}\right)^5$ and in the other $\left(\frac{2-\mu}{2+\mu}\right)^{10}$ is employed to obtain the probability of living through the five or the ten years respectively

Thus, for the age 15–25, $\mu=\cdot00822$

$$\text{so } \frac{2-\cdot00822}{2+\cdot00822}=\frac{1\cdot99178}{2\cdot00822}$$

$$\text{and log. } \left(\frac{1\cdot99178}{2\cdot00822}\right)^{10}=\bar{1}\cdot9643000;$$

which, added to the log. of the number living aged 15 (log. l_{15}) $=5\cdot5374169$, gives log. $l_{25}=5\cdot5017169$; and 317480 is the corresponding number living, aged 25 years (l_{25}).

Dr. Farr gives a table at page clxviii. of his Supplement to the 35th Annual Report of the Registrar-General, comparing the results obtained by this shorter method with those calculated from the same data by interpolation for each age according to the English Life Table, from which it is apparent that the expectation of life by each method up to 15 years is the same; at ages 25 to 65 the differences range from ·37 to ·53 of a year, but after the age of 65 the excess shown by the short method rapidly increases.

In a valuable paper, read before the Statistical Society in April, 1883, on "The Recent Decline in the English Death-rate," **Mr. Noel A. Humphreys** describes a shortened method of constructing a Life Table, and applies it to the years 1876–80. He first of all ascertained the mean annual death-rate in the seventeen years 1838–54, and in the five years 1876–80 at each of the twelve groups of ages given by the Registrar-General in his annual reports. Having then calculated the rate of increase or decrease of the relative rates of the two periods at each group of ages, he started with the annual mortality for males and females respectively *in each year of life*, as given by Dr. Farr's English Life Table No. 3, and raised or lowered these in accordance with the increased or decreased mean mortality prevailing during 1876–80 in the *several groups of ages*. There is an obvious defect in this series of corrected annual rates of mortality which is pointed out by Mr. Humphreys himself. This lies in the assumption that "the changes in the proportions of decrease in the mean rates of succeeding age-periods took place suddenly at the commencement of each period instead of coming gradually into operation, as was certainly the case." But for the purpose of estimating the mean after-lifetime, this method is sufficiently accurate, and forms a comparatively easy method of constructing local Life Tables.

History of Life Tables.—The earliest English Life Table was constructed by **Halley**, the English astronomer, in the second half of the 18th century. It was calculated on the deaths in the city of Breslau in the years 1687–1691. Males and females are not distinguished in it, nor in the Northampton and Carlisle Tables.

De Moivre's hypothesis was suggested by Halley's Breslau tables. He concluded that the hypothesis that out of 86 persons born one dies every year till all are extinct, would very nearly represent the mortality of the greater part of life, and that in the calculation of annuities its errors would nearly compensate one another. Tables formed on this hypothesis, as well as on the Northampton Table to be next considered, overstate the mortality of young adults. The consequence is, that in life assurances calculated on the results of De Moivre's and Price's tables, the young are made to pay for the old, and great injustice is done to those who insure comparatively early in life.

The first Life Table used for the purpose of determining the rate of premium to be paid for Life Assurance was Dr. Price's **Northampton Table**, which was used by the Equitable Office on its establishment in 1762. Like Halley's Table, owing to the want of proper materials, the Northampton Table was not constructed by a comparison of the *deaths and the living at each age*, but from *the deaths alone*. Tables constructed on this latter plan are only correct when the population in which the deaths occur remains stationary; *i.e.*, when the births and deaths are equal in number, and there is no disturbing migration. Dr. Price was under the misapprehension that the population of Northampton was stationary, judging by the number of infantile baptisms. But at the time the data for this Table were recorded, there were a large number of Baptists in Northampton, who repudiated infantile baptism. The consequence of this oversight was that Dr. Price assumed the mean duration of life to be 24 years, when it was really about 30 years. Unfortunately his table was made the basis for the Government annuity schemes; and the same error which gave the insurance offices one-third too high premiums induced the Government to grant annuities by one-third too large for the price charged, resulting in a loss to the public funds of about two millions of money before the error was corrected.

Dr. Price also constructed a correct Life Table from the population and deaths in Sweden, "which was the first national Life Table ever made, and redounds much more to his fame than the Northampton Table" (Farr).

The **Carlisle Table** was formed by Mr. Milne, from the observations of Dr. Heysham, upon the mortality of that town in the years 1779–89, and two enumerations of its population in 1779 and 1787. At the time it was constructed it showed results too favourable for the whole country; but owing to the decrease of mortality which followed, it became more accurate. De Morgan gives the following expression, based on the Carlisle

Table, as representing more nearly the mortality from the age of 15 to that of 65 than does De Moivre's hypothesis. Of every 100 persons, aged 15, one dies every year till the age of 65. Or if we take the mean after-lifetime, according to the Carlisle Table, between the ages of 10 and 60; for rough purposes it may be said: Of persons aged 10 years, the mean after-lifetime is 49 years, with a diminution of 7 years for every 10 years elapsed; thus, of persons aged 20 years, the mean after-lifetime is 49−7=42 years; at 30 years of age, 35 years, and so on. The mean after-lifetime, according to different Life Tables, is shown in the table at page 253.

The differences between the Northampton and Carlisle Tables are seen in the following table, in which are shown the numbers out of 1,000 children born, which, according to these Tables, may be expected to be living at the end of each quinquennial period through life.

Survivors at end of each five years by Northampton and Carlisle Tables.

Age-Groups.	Out of 1,000 Male and Female Children Born.		
	By Northampton Table.	By Carlisle Table.	Difference.
At end of 5 years	536	680	144
„ 10 „	487	646	159
„ 15 „	465	630	165
„ 20 „	441	609	168
„ 25 „	409	588	179
„ 30 „	376	564	188
„ 35 „	344	536	192
„ 40 „	312	508	198
„ 45 „	279	473	194
„ 50 „	245	440	195
„ 55 „	210	407	197
„ 60 „	175	364	189
„ 65 „	140	302	162
„ 70 „	106	240	134
„ 75 „	71	168	97
„ 80 „	40	95	55

Without giving any details respecting the **Amicable Society's Table** and the **Equitable Table**, the latter of which gives the experience of the Equitable Society from 1762 to 1829, of 5,000 lives; or the **Government Tables**, which give the experience of 22,000 government annuitants; or the **Experience Table**, based on the recorded experience of seventeen life offices and 83,905 lives; we must pass on to Dr. Farr's Life Tables, which are based on the census and death-returns of the whole of England and Wales.

English Life Table, No. 1.—Dr. Farr, believing that nothing short of a table based on the returns of the entire kingdom would be satisfactory, constructed his No. 1 table, based on the census returns of 1841 and the deaths of the same year (Registrar-General's 5th Report). Thinking, however, that the records of *one year's deaths* might be open to challenge owing to the short time embraced in them, he recommenced his work, and constructed the **English Life Table, No. 2.** This is founded on the census enumerations of 1831 and 1841, and the deaths of seven years are taken; viz., those in 1841 and the three previous and three subsequent years (Registrar-General's

Number of Males Surviving at end of each Five Years by the English Life Tables.

Age-Groups.	Out of 1,000 Males and Females born.		
	By English Life Table, No. 1.	By English Life Table, No. 2.	By English Life Table, No. 3.
At end of 5 years	373	372	370
" 10 "	355	355	353
" 15 "	345	346	344
" 20 "	333	335	334
" 25 "	319	321	319
" 30 "	304	307	305
" 35 "	288	291	289
" 40 "	271	275	272
" 45 "	253	257	254
" 50 "	233	237	233
" 55 "	213	215	210
" 60 "	188	189	182
" 65 "	155	156	151
" 70 "	118	118	114
" 75 "	78	79	76
" 80 "	43	44	41

12th Annual Report). It is thus based upon the recorded ages of 13,896,797 + 15,914,148 = 29,810,945 persons, and on the registered deaths of 2,436,648 persons.

The difference between these two English Life Tables, as shown by the number of survivors at various ages (page 235), and by the mean after-lifetime, is slight. On the whole, Table No. 2 shows results slightly less favourable to human life than No. 1, for though the number of survivors is greater at most ages in No. 2 than in No. 1 Table, the mean after-lifetime is usually slightly less.

The English Life Table, No. 3, constructed by Dr. Farr, was based on the census enumerations of 1841 and 1851, and upon the 6,470,720 deaths registered in the seventeen years 1838–54. Thus it is not deduced from the population or from the deaths alone, but from the ratio the one bears to the other at different ages, as in the following examples for females:—

Age.	Females.		Annual Rate of Mortality per Unit.
	Living.	Dying in a Year.	
(x)	P_x	d_x	m_x
25 35 45	313,095 281,506 247,434	3,024 3,279 3,555	·00966 ·01165 ·01437

For a detailed description of the methods of construction of this Table, the reader is referred to the "English Life Table, by Dr. W. Farr: Longman & Co, 1864." It consists of three parts, or three Life Tables for (1) persons, (2) males, and (3) females, and each consisting of seven columns. The base of the table for persons is 1,000,000 children born alive; and as boys and girls were born in England during the period of observation in the proportions of 511,745 boys to 488,255 girls, these numbers were made respectively the bases of the male and the female Life Tables. The march of these persons through life is shown in the following diagram, in which

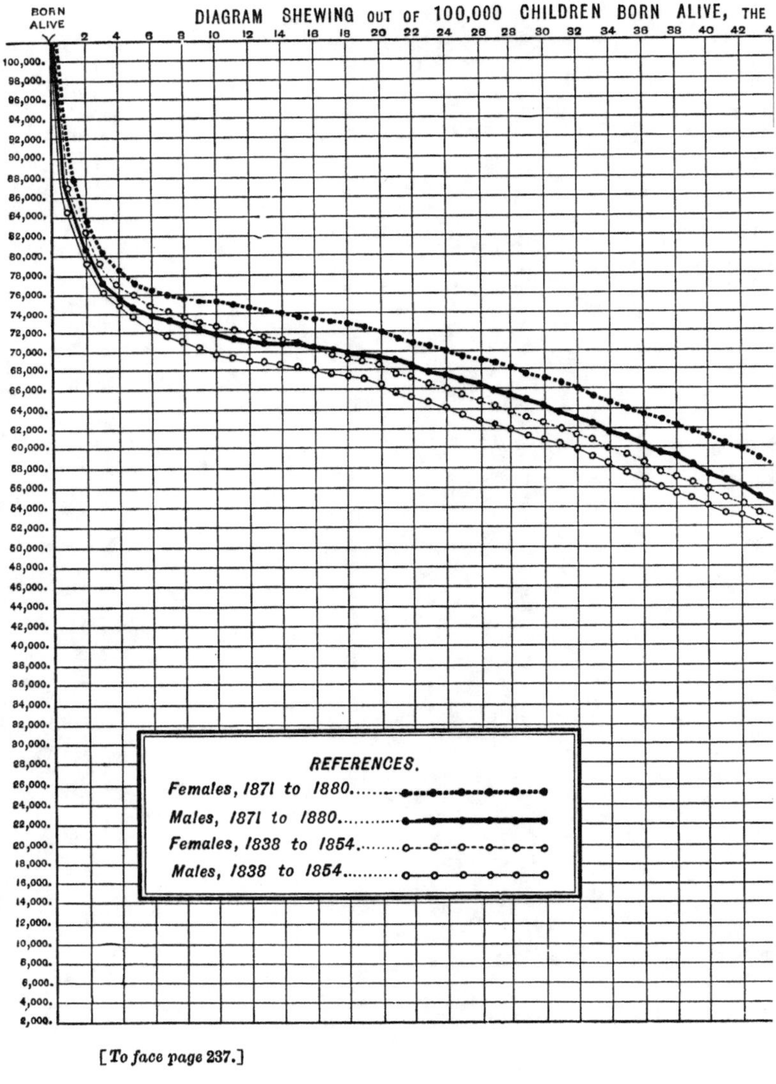

[To face page 237.]

NUMBER THAT SURVIVE TO EACH OF THE UNDERMENTIONED AGES.

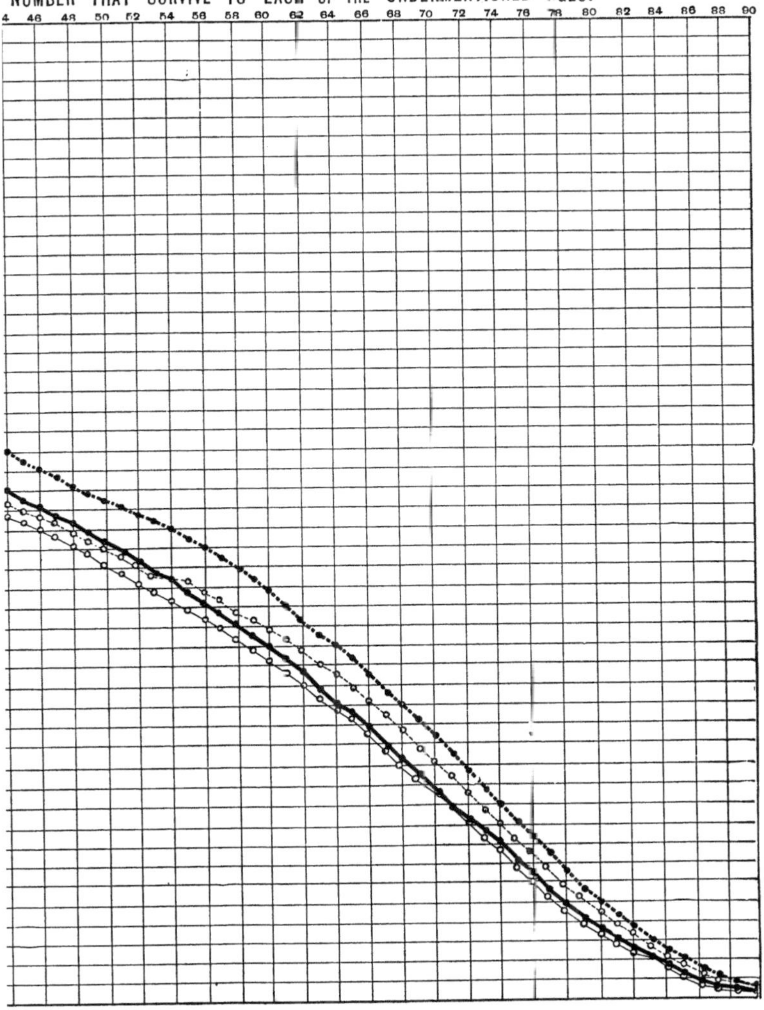

the number of survivors at each age for males and females is given, and compared with the corresponding number in Dr. Ogle's table for 1871–80. It should be noted that in the diagram 100,000 males and the same number of females respectively form the number started with at birth.

The near agreement between the results obtained by these three English Life-Tables is very remarkable, and shows that, spite of annual fluctuations, there was a fairly stationary mortality during 1838–54, which, we may add, continued up to the year 1871. The latter fact led Dr. Farr to abandon his intention of constructing a fourth English Life-Table down to 1872.

The **Healthy Districts Life-Table** was constructed by Dr. Farr on the basis of the mortality during the five years 1849–53, in 63 selected English districts which showed, during the decennium 1841–50, a mean annual death-rate not exceeding 17 per 1,000 persons living. As pointed out by Dr. Farr, it expresses "very accurately the actual duration of life among the clergy and other classes of the community living under favourable circumstances." It represents also a standard of healthiness already attained, and is therefore useful for purposes of comparison. This table is printed in the 33rd Annual Report of the Registrar-General.

The **Upper Class Experience Table** was constructed by Mr. C. Ansell from data collected by him as to men of the upper and professional classes, and given in his "Statistics of Families in the Upper and Professional Classes."

The **Healthy Males Table** given in the following table is the healthy males table of the Institute of Actuaries, and is based on the experience of the principal insurance offices in regard to insured, and therefore exceptionally healthy, lives.

The **Clerical Experience Table** is based on data respecting over 5,000 clergymen living between 1760 and 1860.

The **New English Life-Table** by Dr. Ogle, published in the supplement to the 35th Annual Report of the Registrar-General, starts with a million males and a million females, and shows the number surviving at each age (see chart facing this page) and the mean expectation of life at each age (page 238).

Comparative View of Number of Survivors at Different Ages according to various Life Tables. (Ogle.)

Age.	Life Table.	Percentage of Males that Survive												
		5 years.	10 years.	15 years.	20 years.	25 years.	30 years.	35 years.	40 years.	45 years.	50 years.	55 years.	60 years.	65 years.
10	New English. . . .	98	96	93	89	84	79	74	67	60	51	42	31	20
	Old ,, ...	98	94	90	86	82	77	72	66	59	52	43	32	21
	Healthy Males . . .	98	96	93	90	86	82	78	73	67	59	49	38	26
	Healthy Districts . .	98	96	92	89	85	81	77	73	68	62	53	43	30
	Upper Class Experience	98	95	91	87	83	79	75	70	65	59	51	43	?
	Clerical	—	—	—	—	—	—	—	—	—	—	—	—	
15	New English. . . .	98	94	90	86	81	75	68	61	52	43	32	21	
	Old ,, ...	97	93	88	84	79	74	68	61	53	44	33	22	
	Healthy Males . . .	98	95	91	88	84	79	74	68	60	50	39	26	
	Healthy Districts . .	97	94	90	86	83	79	74	69	63	54	43	31	
	Upper Class Experience	97	93	88	84	80	76	71	66	60	52	43	?	
	Clerical	—	—	—	—	—	—	—	—	—	—	—		
20	New English. . . .	97	93	88	83	77	70	62	54	44	33	21		
	Old ,, ...	96	91	87	82	76	70	63	55	45	34	23		
	Healthy Males . . .	97	93	90	86	81	76	69	61	51	40	27		
	Healthy Districts . .	96	93	89	85	81	76	71	65	56	45	32		
	Upper Class Experience	96	91	87	83	78	73	68	62	54	45	?		
	Clerical	—	—	—	—	—	—	—	—	—	—			
25	New English. . . .	96	91	86	79	73	65	56	45	34	22			
	Old ,, ...	95	90	85	79	73	66	57	47	36	24			
	Healthy Males . . .	97	93	88	84	78	71	63	53	41	28			
	Healthy Districts . .	96	92	88	84	79	74	67	58	46	33			
	Upper Class Experience	95	91	86	82	76	71	65	56	47	?			
	Clerical	97	94	91	87	82	76	68	58	46	33			
30	New English. . . .	95	89	83	76	67	58	47	35	23				
	Old ,, ...	95	89	83	77	69	60	49	38	25				
	Healthy Males . . .	96	92	87	81	74	66	55	42	29				
	Healthy Districts . .	96	92	87	82	77	70	60	48	34				
	Upper Class Experience	95	91	86	80	75	70	59	49	?				
	Clerical	97	94	90	85	78	70	60	47	34				
35	New English. . . .	94	87	80	71	61	50	37	24					
	Old ,, ...	94	88	81	73	63	52	40	26					
	Healthy Males . . .	95	90	84	77	68	57	44	30					
	Healthy Districts . .	96	91	86	80	73	63	50	35					
	Upper Class Experience	95	90	84	79	71	62	51	?					
	Clerical	96	92	87	81	72	62	49	35					

Continued,—

Age.	Life Table.	Percentage of Males that Survive												
		5 years.	10 years.	15 years.	20 years.	25 years.	30 years.	35 years.	40 years.	45 years.	50 years.	55 years.	60 years.	65 years.
40	New English. . . .	93	85	75	65	53	39	26						
	Old ,, ...	93	86	77	67	55	42	28						
	Healthy Males . . .	95	88	81	72	60	46	31						
	Healthy Districts . .	95	90	84	76	66	53	37						
	Upper Class Experience	95	88	83	75	65	54	?						
	Clerical	96	90	83	75	64	51	36						
45	New English. . . .	91	81	70	57	43	28							
	Old ,, ...	92	83	72	59	45	30							
	Healthy Males . . .	93	85	76	63	49	33							
	Healthy Districts . .	94	88	80	69	55	39							
	Upper Class Experience	93	87	79	69	57	?							
	Clerical	94	87	78	67	53	38							
50	New English. . . .	89	77	62	47	30								
	Old ,, ...	90	78	65	49	32								
	Healthy Males . . .	91	81	68	52	35								
	Healthy Districts . .	93	85	73	59	42								
	Upper Class Experience	94	85	74	61	?								
	Clerical	92	83	71	56	40								
55	New English. . . .	86	70	52	34									
	Old ,, ...	87	72	55	36									
	Healthy Males . . .	88	74	57	39									
	Healthy Districts . .	91	79	63	45									
	Upper Class Experience	91	79	65	?									
	Clerical	90	77	61	43									
60	New English. . . .	81	61	40										
	Old ,, ...	83	63	42										
	Healthy Males . . .	84	65	44										
	Healthy Districts . .	86	69	49										
	Upper Class Experience	87	72	?										
	Clerical	85	68	48										
65	New English. . . .	75	49											
	Old ,, ...	76	50											
	Healthy Males . . .	77	52											
	Healthy Districts . .	80	57											
	Upper Class Experience	83	?											
	Clerical	79	56											
70	New English. . . .	65												
	Old ,, ...	66												
	Healthy Males . . .	67												
	Healthy Districts . .	71												
	Upper Class Experience	?												
	Clerical	71												

From this valuable table, arranged by Dr. W. Ogle (*Journal of the Statistical Society*, vol. vii. pt. iv. page 640), a comparison can readily be made between several Life Tables based on the mortality of males, and the influence of social or other conditions on vitality can be approximately estimated.

The ages to which the percentages apply are given in the first vertical column to the left of the page, and the percentage of males surviving 5, 10, 15, etc., years, according to the several Life Tables are given in the horizontal columns.

The comparison between the old and new English Tables shows that in 1838–54 the chances of life were less favourable at the younger ages, and more favourable at the older ages, than in 1871-80. For instance, of 100 children just ten years old, 86 would survive 20 years by the old table, and 82 by the new Table ; but after an interval of 50 years (*i.e.*, at 60 years of age) 52 would survive by the old, and 51 by the new table.

The Healthy Males Table being founded on insured and therefore selected lives, shows a considerably larger percentage of survivals throughout than does the English Life Table.

A comparison of the upper-class experience table with the old English Life Table shows the effect of more favourable social circumstances; and were the figures for ages under 10 given, the comparison would be much more in favour of the upper-class table. For short periods the chances of survival are not widely different ; but when the chances of survival for longer periods are considered, the differences are very great. Thus, of 100 children just 10 years old, 32 live 60 years longer by the old English Life Table, and 43 by the upper-class table ; and of 100 men 55 years old, 87 are alive after 5 years interval by the English Table, and 91 by the upper-class table.

In comparing the clerical experience table with the upper-class table, the advantage is largely on the side of the clergy in all the periods of life, except for the later ages or for long survivals. It is not easy to see any satisfactory explanation of this, and Dr. Ogle suspects that one or other of these tables has been based on too small a number of observations.

CHAPTER XV.

THE DURATION OF LIFE.

Connection between Mean Age at Death, Expectation of Life, and Number out of which One Dies Annually.—Mean Age at Death.—Effect of Birth-Rate on Mean Age at Death.—Mean Age at Death from Certain Diseases.—Mean Age of Living.—Mean Duration of Life.—Complete and Curtate Expectation of Life.—Willich's and Farr's Formulæ.—Probable Duration of Life.—Specific Intensity.—Probability of Living a given Number of Years.—Probability of Dying of any one Disease.

THE duration of life is the problem with which Vital Statistics are largely occupied. As Babbage has put it, "Nothing is more uncertain than the duration of life when the maxim is applied to the individual; but there are few things less subject to fluctuation than the duration of life in a multitude of individuals." It is on this principle that annuities and life assurances can be made the subject of definite and exact calculations, the final results being found to vary within very narrow limits.

Several tests are employed to measure the duration of human life, and we are at present concerned to determine their precise value, and the relationship existing between them.

Those most commonly employed are:—

(1) The mean age at death;
(2) The probable duration of life;
(3) The mean duration of life;
(4) The expectation of life, or mean after-lifetime;
(5) The number living out of which one dies annually.

Before discussing the value of these different tests of vitality, the student should understand the close relationship (amounting to numerical identity) which exists between the mean age at death, the expectation of life, and the number out of which one dies annually, in a Life-Table or normal population.

In a Life Table, of which an elementary specimen is shown below, it is evident that the number against any age in the

Age.	Number who	
	Completed that year, l_x.	Died in their next year, d_x.
Col. 1.	Col. 2.	Col. 3.
0	10,000	1,495
1	8,505	537
3	7,968	282
4	7,501	185
5	7,368	133
6	7,269	99
7	7,191	78
8	7,126	55
9	7,071	46
10	7,025	40
...	...	...
...	...	...
...	...	...
94	31	10
95	22	7
96	14	6
97	9	4
98	6	3
99	4	1
100	2	0

second column is equal to the sum of those in the third column against that and all the greater ages; from which we infer that the number who *complete* any year of age is equal to the sum of those dying at all the greater ages. Thus in the table, the number who annually complete their ninety-sixth year (=14) is equal to the sum of the annual deaths at all the greater ages. On the assumption that the deaths in any year are distributed at equal intervals in the year, it follows that the number living in any year of their age, such as would be ascertained in a census enumeration, is an arithmetical mean between the number entering upon and the number completing that year.

Thus it appears that—

The number of the living in their	Is half the sum of
95th year	31 and 22
96th ,,	22 ,, 14
97th ,,	14 ,, 9
98th ,,	9 ,, 6
99th ,,	6 ,, 4
100th ,,	4 ,, 2
101st ,,	2 ,, 0

It will be observed, however, that the same numbers occur in each of these two series, with the exception of 31 and 0, the first and the last. Therefore the sum of the second series falls short of the sum of the first by 31, and the series of half sums or means would fall short of the sum of the first series by $\frac{31}{2}$. The same reasoning would apply for any other age. It follows then that the number of persons living at any age x and upwards, is less than the sum of the numbers annually completing that and all the greater ages by half the number who annually complete the age x.

Now in the elementary Life Table just given, if the sum of the numbers living at any age x and all greater ages be taken (in column 2), *each life is counted once for every complete year it survives after the age x.* Thus on the supposition that the average duration of existence during any year of age for those who die during that year is half a year, it follows that if we add to the sum of the numbers living at the age x and all greater ages half the number marked in column 2 as living at the age x, the sum total thus obtained will evidently be the whole duration of life after the age x, enjoyed by all the lives who survive the age x on the Life Table.

If this sum total be divided by the number who by the life-table annually survive this age, the quotient will be the individual expectation of life after the age x.

But we have seen that this sum total is also the number constantly living in the place, at and above the age x. Hence the expectation of life after the age x is obtained by dividing the number living at and above the age x by the number who annually complete that age. If the number constantly living at *all* ages be divided by the number of annual *births* or *deaths*, the expectation of life at birth is obtained. But the sum of the numbers living at the age x and all higher ages represents the entire population at and above the age x; and inasmuch as these all die at this or some subsequent age, if this sum be divided by the number living at the age x, we obtain the number out of which one dies annually. Consequently in a Life-Table population the expectation of life at any age is equal to the number of living persons of that age and upwards out of which one dies annually.

In Dr. Farr's Life-Table population, the persons become reduced to one-half in 45 years = the probable lifetime; the mean after-lifetime = 40·9 years, or very nearly 41 years; and this = the mean age at death. To forty-one persons living there is one birth and one death annually; the rate of mortality is one in forty-one; and forty-one is the mean duration of life.

Mean Age at Death $= \dfrac{\text{sum of ages at death}}{\text{number of deaths}}$. Thus if five persons die at the ages 10, 20, 30, 40, 50, their mean age at death $= \dfrac{10+20+30+40+50}{5} = 30$ years; and if a second group of five die at the age of 25, 30, 45, 50, 70 respectively, their mean age at death will be $\dfrac{25+30+45+50+70}{5} = 44$ years. Assuming that these two groups of persons were exposed during life to similar influences, the question arises, Would the mean age at death of the two groups form a safe standard of comparison between them? It should be noted, to begin with, that the number of persons in the instances quoted is very small, and cannot therefore form a trustworthy basis for comparison. But even if each group embraced a large number of persons, erroneous conclusions would certainly be drawn, unless the special circumstances and age-constitution of each group were identical. In a normal or Life-Table population, the mean age at death is the same as the expectation of life at birth (mean lifetime). But in a population like that of England and Wales, where the births constantly exceed the deaths, the mean age at death is low, apart altogether from any low sanitary status. Similarly in a population subject to migration, as is that of England to an enormous extent, unless it can be shown that immigrants are of the same age as emigrants or deceased persons, the mean age at death will not furnish a trustworthy measure of the true duration of life.

By the English Life Table, No. 3, the mean age at death is 40·9 years. But during the seventeen years, 1838–54, in addition to the 380,631 annual births to balance the 380,631 deaths, 191,068 more children were born annually, making a total annual addition of 571,699 children to the population. Consequently the mean age of all dying in these seventeen years was 29·4 instead of 40·9, the 11·5 years' difference being the result of the excess of young lives.

Thus (1) in *contrasting different nations*, the mean age at death is a most fallacious test. Dr. Guy takes as an instance two populations, A having 46 per cent. of its population under twenty years old, and B having 54 per cent. under twenty years old; the proportions above twenty being reversed. Now about half the inhabitants in A and B die under twenty, and if the mean age at death of these be assumed to be five years, and of all over twenty to be sixty years, then the mean age at death of fifty persons

$$\text{in } A=\frac{46}{2}\times 5+\frac{54}{2}\times 60=115+1620=1735\,;$$

$$\text{in } B=\frac{54}{2}\times 5+\frac{46}{2}\times 60=135+1380=1515.$$

$$\text{Therefore the mean age at death in A}=\frac{1735}{50}=34{\cdot}7 \text{ years.}$$

$$\text{in } B=\frac{1515}{50}=30{\cdot}3 \text{ years.}$$

Thus, on the assumption that the general death-rate in A and B is the same, the mean age at death differs by 4·4 years, owing to varying age-composition of the two populations. In the following table (Farr's "Vital Statistics," page 473), it will be observed that in England, where the mean age at death was lowest of three countries in 1841, the mortality was also lowest, but the true expectation of life, as deduced from a Life Table, was highest; whereas if the mean age at death were a trustworthy test of the duration of life, a low mean age at death ought to be accompanied by a high mortality.

	Mortality; or, One Death.	Mean Age at Death.	Mean After-lifetime or Expectation of Life.
England (1841)	In 46 living	29 years	41 years
France "	" 42 "	34 "	40 " ?
Sweden "	" 41 "	31 "	39 "
Metropolis "	" 41 "	29 "	37 "
Liverpool "	" 30 "	21 "	26 "
Surrey (extra-Metropolitan)	" 52 "	34 "	45 "

It may be inferred from the above table that the mortality number out of which one death occurs), although it does not pretend to express the true mean duration of life (expectation of life), gives a much nearer approximation to it than does the mean age at death. This will be at once seen if the mortality and expectation of life columns in the preceding table be arranged side by side, for they coincide in position in every instance, unlike the mean age at death, which gives very variable indications.

(2) In contrasting the *same country at different periods*, similar fallacies may arise. As shown by Mr. Neison in the 7th vol. of the "Journal of Statistical Society," 49 per cent. of the total population was under twenty in England in 1821, but in 1841 only 46 per cent., which would have considerable effect on the mean age at death.

(3) We have seen that *urban populations* consist in a much larger proportion of persons under forty than do *rural* populations. Similar differences may exist between the several

districts of large cities, and correction for different age-constitution of populations may sometimes reverse the apparent position of the populations under comparison.

(4) In the comparison of different *classes of society*, and those engaged in different *occupations*, serious errors have arisen by the incautious use of this test to determine their relative sanitary condition. It would be absurd, for instance, to draw any inferences from a comparison of the mean ages at death of bishops and curates, as men do not usually become bishops till they have passed the middle period of life. Similarly in comparing the gentry with tradesmen. Most of the gentry are retired tradesmen, and their mean age at death is therefore higher than that of tradesmen. The low mean age at death of dressmakers has been adduced as a proof of the unhealthy character of their employment. Without denying the latter fact, the low mean age at death of dressmakers is no more a proof of their insanitary circumstances than is a low mean age at death among the pupils in a boarding school.

The use of the mean age at death as a test of the sanitary condition of different classes is only justifiable when the age and sex constitution of those living in the classes compared is the same. If only a section of a class is taken, then this section must be uniform in age and sex constitution with the section of another class, with which comparison is instituted.

The acceptance of the mean age at death as a test of the duration of life is a fragment of the error involved in the construction of a Life Table from the deaths alone, as in Dr. Price's Northampton Table. When a population remains stationary for a long series of years, the mean age at death of such a population is equivalent to the true duration of life, and Dr. Price chose a population which he believed to be stationary. But the Northampton population was not stationary, and consequently the Northampton Table did not give a true estimate of the duration of life.

Effect of the Birth-rate upon the Mean Age at Death.—We have already seen that in a stationary population the mean duration of life (or expectation of life at birth) is identical with the mean age at death, and with the number of the population out of which one death annually occurs; or, inasmuch as the births and deaths are equal in number, the number out of which one annual birth occurs. But if a population is not stationary, the state of matters is altogether different.

Dr. Richardson claimed for the inhabitants of his "Hygeiopolis," that their death-rate would be reduced to five per 1,000. It was soon afterwards asserted in the *Times* that this would imply a mean duration of life (using the term in the sense of mean age at death) of 200 years, and that *a fortiori* Dr. Richardson's anticipations were absurd. It is only, however, where the population is stationary that the mean age at death would be 200 years, the deficiency of those who live a shorter time being balanced by the excess of those who live a longer time.

Dr. Bristowe, in the St. Thomas's Hospital Report for 1876, has worked out the influence of variations in the birth and death-rate on the mean age at death. He assumes the simplest condition of things, viz., that in each case the birth-rate and death-rate continue uniform from year to year; that no immigration or emigration occurs; and that every individual born into the population attains the mean age, or, in other words, all the inhabitants die at the same age. Under these conditions three cases present themselves:—

(1) Where the births exceed the deaths;

(2) Where the two are equal, and the population is stationary;

(3) Where the deaths exceed the births and the population progressively decreases.

In the first case, the population, births and deaths all increase from year to year by geometrical progression.

Let number of population from which we start $=1$, and $b=$ birth-rate, and $d=$death-rate of this unit, and $r=$its annual increase; *i.e.*, $r=b-d$.

Then the following three series will represent the annual growth of the population, of the births, and of the deaths respectively.

	Population.	Births.	Deaths.
1st Year . .	1 . .	b . .	d
2nd „ . .	$(1+r)$ . .	$b\,(1+r)$ . .	$d(1+r)$
3rd „ . .	$(1+r)^2$ . .	$b\,(1+r)^2$ . .	$d\,(1+r)^2$
4th „ . .	$(1+r)^3$ . .	$b\,(1+r)^3$ . .	$d\,(1+r)^3$
nth „ . .	$(1+r)^{n-1}$ . .	$b\,(1+r)^{n-1}$ . .	$d\,(1+r)^{n-1}$

According to the hypothesis with which we started, all the persons born in any one year die together in the course of some subsequent year, and the number of that year, reckoning from the time of births, is the mean age at death. It is evident, therefore, that if we can ascertain the number of that term in which $d\,(1+r)^{n-1}=b$, the value of the index n–1 will represent the mean age at death. Let $x=$the value of the unknown index.

Now from $d\,(1+r)^x=b$, we obtain

$$(1+r)^x=\frac{b}{d},$$

and taking the log. of each side of this equation,

$$x\log.\,(1+r)=\log.\,b-\log.\,d$$

$$\therefore\ x=\frac{\log.\,b-\log.\,d}{\log.\,(1+r)}$$

from which equation the value of x is easily determined.

In the second case in which $b=d$, the above equation is useless, inasmuch as $r=o$, and the equation will become $n=\frac{\log.\,1}{\log.\,1}=0$, the value of which is indeterminate.

In the third case, in which d is greater than b, and r becomes a negative quantity, we have a diminishing series in geometrical progression.

The assumptions made as to the constitution of the population and their uniform age at death are absent in experience; hence we must expect that the results obtained by the above formula, when applied to an ordinary population, will only approximate to the truth. They serve, however, to show that a high death-rate is compatible with longevity, and *vice versâ;*

also that a low death-rate, apart from all considerations as to the birth-rate, does not necessarily imply a long-lived population. Dr. Bristowe calculated a large table for varying values of b and d, showing that with d as low as ·005 (5 per 1,000), the mean age at death varies from 7·6 years when $b=1·005$, to 200 when $b=·005$, and 510 when $b=·0005$; and with $d=·04$ it varied from 4·7 when $b=1·04$, to 25 when $b=·04$ and 108 when $b=·0005$.

The **mean age at death from certain diseases** is of considerable interest from a medical standpoint. Some causes of death are almost confined to the first year of life, as premature birth, atrophy, convulsions, teething; others belong chiefly to the old, as cancer and paralysis; while childbirth, fever, and phthisis are most fatal in the middle period of life.

In the following table the mean age at death from various diseases for males and females separately is displayed.

Mean Age at Death of Males and Females who Died from Certain Diseases in the 25 *years*, 1848–72.

Causes of Death.	Mean Age at Death.		
	Males.	Females.	Mean.
All Causes	28·2	30·8	29·5
Whooping Cough . .	1·7	1·8	1·8
Measles	2·5	2·8	2·7
Croup	3·1	3·2	3·2
Diphtheria (1859–72) .	7·7	8·1	7·9
Scarlet Fever (1859–72)	5·2	5·6	5·4
Smallpox	13·2	10·6	11·9
Diarrhœa	11·8	14·9	13·4
Typhus	26·6	25·4	26·0
Cholera	30·4	32·4	31·4
Erysipelas	35·7	32·8	34·3
Rheumatism	39·8	41·4	40·6
Influenza	42·8	48·8	45·8
Carbuncle	59·2	57·9	58·6

A statement of the number of deaths from different diseases in proportion to total deaths is unreliable as an indication of their relative prevalence, the proportion of deaths from diseases of the young being overstated in an increasing population such as that of England. The true proportions can be shown only by a Life Table.

If the following table is examined (from Supplement to 35th Annual Report of Registrar-General, p. xxvii.), it will be seen that, owing to the excess of young people in the English population, the death-rate per million of the population living at all ages is overstated in the case of smallpox, scarlet fever, measles, whooping cough, and, in fact, all diseases of the young; whereas the mortality from childbirth and fever (occurring at ages near the mean age of the living population) is undisturbed. The constitution of the population should be taken into account in comparing the death-rate from any given disease with the corresponding death-rate of another country, in which the population may be more nearly stationary than in England.

Mean Age at Death of Persons Dying from Certain Diseases, 1848–72; *also Proportion to Deaths from All Causes, and Rates of Mortality.*

Cause of Death.	Mean Age at Death 1848–72.	Deaths to 1,000,000 Deaths from all Causes Deduced from		Annual Rate of Mortality to 1,000,000 Living of all Ages Deduced from	
		Life Table.	Registered Deaths.	Life Table.	Registered Deaths.
Whooping Cough	1·8	15,161	23,145	371	521
Measles. . . .	2·7	12,865	19,134	315	437
Scarlet Fever and Diphtheria. .	5·8	34,966	48,247	856	1,046
Smallpox . . .	11·9	6,521	8,535	160	204
Typhus. . . .	26·0	38,107	40,170	933	918
Childbirth and Metria . . .	31·7	6,921	7,364	169	168

Dr. Rumsey has urged that returns should be made of the

$$\textbf{mean age of the living} = \frac{\text{sum of ages of population at census}}{\text{number of population}}$$

as a corrective of the fallacies connected with the mean age at death. Mr. Chadwick found that in fairly healthy districts the mean age of the living was to the mean age at death as about 3 to 4, while in insanitary districts with shifting and increasing populations the line of vitality was higher than that of mortality. But this is due to the fact that under insanitary conditions a high mortality spends itself chiefly among young children, and, in addition, there are always crowds of young and healthy persons ready to immigrate from country to town, thus lowering the mean age of the town populations, among whom insanitary conditions are especially rife. On the whole, therefore, the mean age of the living as a test of the duration of life is as untrustworthy as is the mean age of the dying.

The **Mean Duration of Life**, or *vie moyenne*, when a population is stationary in numbers and is not disturbed by migration, or other causes,—when, in other words, its age and sex constitution do not alter,—is, if we start with birth, identical with the mean age at death, and with the expectation of life as found by a Life Table. It is also, under the same circumstances, identical with the mortality as expressed by the number living out of which one death occurs.

Thus, in a stationary population,—

$$\left.\begin{array}{l}\text{Mean Age at Death}\\ \text{Mean Duration of Life}\\ \text{Expectation of Life}\end{array}\ \text{at birth}\right\} = \frac{\text{No. of Population}}{\text{No. of Deaths in one Year}}$$

$$= \frac{\text{Sum of Ages at Death}}{\text{Total No. of Deaths}}$$

When the population is not stationary, the mean duration of life has the same signification as the mean after-lifetime from birth next to be considered. During the decennium 1871–80, the mean age at death for males in England and Wales was 29 years; the mean duration of life was 41·35 years, while 1 in 44·2 died annually, instead of these three figures being identical, as they would have been had the population been stationary. The mean duration of life for the years after birth will be explained when we have considered the expectation of life.

The **Expectation of Life** (also called the mean after-life-time) is found from a Life Table, constructed on the basis of the number living and the number dying at each age. Such a Life Table shows how many of a given number started with live through each year of subsequent life, and what is the sum of the number of years they live. The expectation of life is obtained by dividing the sum of these years by the number living at the year of age for which the expectation of life is desired.

The expectation of life at different ages and according to different Life Tables is shown in the following table:—

Expectation of Life (Mean After-lifetime) according to various Life Tables at successive ages.

Years of Age.	De Moivre's Hypothesis.	Northampton Table.	Carlisle Table.	English Life Table, No 1.	English Life Table, No 2.	English Life Table, No. 3.		New English Life Table (Ogle).	
	Persons.					Males.	Females.	Males.	Females.
0	43·	25·2	38·7	41·1	—	39·91	41·85	41·35	44·62
5	40·5	40·8	51·3	50·0	—	49·71	50·33	50·87	53·08
10	38·	39·8	48·8	47·2	47·5	47·05	47·67	47·60	49·76
15	35 5	36·5	45·0	43·6	43·4	43·18	43·90	43·41	45·63
20	33·	33·4	41 5	40·3	40 0	39·48	40·29	39·40	41·66
25	30·5	30·9	37 9	37·0	36·6	36·12	37·04	35·68	37·98
30	28·	28·3	34 3	33·6	33·1	32·76	33·81	32·10	34·41
35	25·5	25·7	31·0	30·4	29·8	29·40	30·59	28·64	30·90
40	23·	23·1	27·6	27·1	26·5	26·06	27·34	25·30	27·46
45	20·5	20·5	24·5	23·8	23·1	22·76	24·06	22·07	24·06
50	18·	18·0	21·1	20·6	19·9	19·54	20·75	18·93	20·68
55	15·5	15·6	17·6	17·1	16·7	16·45	17·43	15·95	17·33
60	13·	13·2	14·3	14·0	13·6	13·53	14·34	13·14	14·24
65	10·5	10·9	11·8	11·1	10·9	10·82	11·51	10·55	11·42
70	8·	8·6	9·2	8·7	8·6	8·45	9·02	8·27	8·95
75	5·5	6·5	7·0	6·7	6·6	6·49	6·93	6.34	6·87
80	3·	4·8	5·5	5·1	5·0	4·93	5·26	4·79	5·20
85	0·5	3·4	4·1	3·7	3·7	3·73	3·98	3·56	3·88
90	—	2·4	3·3	2·7	—	2·84	3·01	2·66	2·90
95	—	0·8	3·5	2·1	—	2·17	2·29	2·01	2·17
100	—	—	2·3	—	—	1·68	1·76	1·61	1·62

It should be observed that the expectation of life is the

average number of years which persons of a given age, taken one with another, live, assuming that they die according to a given table of the probabilities of life. The term "expectation of life" does not imply that an individval may reasonably expect to live a given number of years. The excess of those who die late is distributed among those who die early, "those who live longer enjoying as much more in proportion to their number, as those who fall short enjoy less of life." Thus the expectation of life has no relation whatever to the most probable lifetime of any given individual.

In actuarial language, a **complete** and a **curtate expectation of life** are described. The relation between these, at the risk of some repetition, may be briefly stated as follows (see also page 229):—

Let l_x = number of persons living at age x, and l_{x+1} the number living at the end of an additional year. Then these l_{x+1} persons will have each lived a complete year in the first year, or among them l_{x+1} complete years. Similarly l_{x+2} will live another complete year each in the second year, or among them a further l_{x+2} complete years, and so on for future years. The total number of complete years lived by l_x persons until they become extinct will therefore be—

$$l_{x+1} + l_{x+2} + l_{x+3} + l_{x+4} + \text{etc.} + \text{etc.};$$

giving for each of the l_x persons an average number of complete years, $\dfrac{l_{x+1} + l_{x+2} + l_{x+3} + \text{etc.}}{l_x}$.

This average number of complete years lived by l_x persons is called the *Curtate Expectation of Life* at age x and $= e_x$.

We have, however, in the above confined our attention to the complete years of life, and have not taken into account that portion of lifetime lived by each person in the year of his death. In some instances this may be only a few days, in others nearly an entire year; but it may be assumed, with a fair degree of accuracy, taking one person with another, that l_x persons will live in the aggregate $\frac{1}{2} l_x$ years in the year of death, or an average of half a year for each.

If we add this half year to the curtate expectation of life, we obtain the *Complete Expectation of Life*, which is equal to

$$\tfrac{1}{2} + \frac{l_{x+1} + l_{x+2} + l_{x+3} + \text{etc.}}{l_x} = \mathring{e}_x.$$

The rule, then, for obtaining the complete expectation of life is to divide the sum of the number who complete each age above the given one by the number living at the given age, and then to the quotient add half-unity.

Having given the expectation of life, it is easy to find *the true* or mean duration of life, which is the present age added to the expectation of life. Thus at birth the expectation of life and mean duration of life are identical; at the age x the expectation of life being $\mathring{e}_x$; the mean duration of life of l_x persons will be $x + \mathring{e}_x$. Thus by the English Life Table No. 3 the female expectation of life at the age of 20 years is 40·81 years; therefore the mean duration of life for women aged 20 is 60·81 years. It will be seen that the true mean duration of life differs from the mean age at death, in that the former is a calculation based on all the deaths occurring after a given age, in the members of a population traced through life; while the latter is a calculation based on such deaths as happen to be noted in a population continually disturbed by births, immigration and emigration.

It should be noted that by many writers the term *mean duration of life* is used as absolutely synonymous with expectation of life for all ages, instead of signifying, as we have employed it, the present age in years *plus* the expectation of life. At birth the two terms are in any case synonymous. Dr. Farr and Mr. Milne used the two terms as having the same signification throughout, and this must be remembered in the following quotations from Mr. Milne, which point out the relation between duration of life and mortality: "When the population has been increasing, the mean duration of life, according to the table, will be less than the number out of which one person dies annually in that population, but *the difference will be small* except under particular circumstances;'

while the mean age at which persons die "will fall short of the number of the people out of which one dies annually *by a much greater number.*" Thus "when the proportion of the people dying annually is known, it will not be difficult to judge whether a table of mortality (Life Table) for that people has been constructed properly from the necessary data; or, what is much more common and more easily effected, by summation of the deaths at all ages." Mr. Milne also points out that in an increasing population the mean age at death is lower, and the annual mortality less, than in a stationary population having the same expectation of life. This is owing to the fact that the increase of the population causes an excess of persons between 5 and 55, among whom the mortality is lower than among persons of all ages.

In cases where a Life Table is unobtainable, the **formula of Willich** gives approximate results, not very far from the truth, for ages between 25 and 75. It is as follows:—

If x = expectation of life, and a = present age, then $x = \frac{2}{3}(80 - a)$.

Thus at the age of 40 years the expectation of life according to this formula $= \frac{2}{3}(80-40) = 26{\cdot}7$ years. By the English Life Table No. 3, the expectation of life for this age is 26·06 years for males and 27·34 years for females.

Dr. Farr gives another **formula**, by means of which an approximation to the expectation of life at birth may be obtained, when the birth- and death-rates are known.

If b = birth-rate and d = death-rate per unit of population, then expectation of life $= \left(\frac{2}{3} \times \frac{1}{d}\right) + \left(\frac{1}{3} \times \frac{1}{b}\right)$.

Thus, in the decennium 1871–80, the birth-rate was 35·45 per 1,000 = ·03545 per unit, and the death-rate 21·4 per 1,000 = ·0214 per unit.

The expectation of life $= \left(\frac{2}{3} \times \frac{1}{\cdot 0214}\right) + \left(\frac{1}{3} \times \frac{1}{\cdot 03535}\right) = 43{\cdot}63$ years.

By Dr. Ogle's Life Table for the corresponding period, the expectation of life for males was 41·35, and for females 44·62 years.

The **Probable Duration of Life** (also called equation of life, or *vie probable*) is a term used to signify the age at which any number of children born into the world will be reduced to one-half, so that there are equal chances of their dying before and after that age. The name is unfortunate, as every possible duration of life has a probability which may be determined, and is therefore mathematically a "probable lifetime." Using the term, however, in its limited sense, it will be seen from the following table that at birth the probable duration of life is in excess of the expectation of life, and continues so in a gradually decreasing amount until after the age of 50, when the conditions are reversed. The 511,745 boys at birth who form the basis of the table become reduced to one-half by the time they reach their forty-fifth year; and the 488,255 girls who form the basis of the table lose half their number by the forty-seventh year.

The Probable Lifetime (Vie Probable) and the After-lifetime (Vie Moyenne) according to the English Life Table No. 3.

Age.	Males.		Females.	
	Probable Lifetime.	After-lifetime.	Probable Lifetime.	After-lifetime.
0	44·43	39·91	46·42	41·85
10	50·98	47·05	52·29	47·67
20	42·55	39·48	44·00	40·29
30	34·77	32·76	36·32	33·81
40	27·09	26·06	28·68	27·34
50	19·71	19·54	21·08	20·75
60	13·00	13·53	13·91	14·34
70	7·55	8·15	8·15	9·02
80	4·04	4·93	4·37	5·26
90	2·20	2·84	2·35	3·01
99	1·36	1·76	1·44	1·86

The probable duration of life is simply the age at which a

given population is reduced by one-half its number. It must not be regarded as representing any actual fact for individuals, inasmuch as the mortality is most unevenly distributed, the deaths being concentrated at certain periods of life with comparative blanks in between. De Moivre assumed that the decrements of population are in arithmetical progression, and that of every 86 persons born, one would die uniformly every year until all were extinct. Such an assumption was convenient in the calculation of annuity tables, before accurate Life Tables were constructed. According to this hypothesis, there is no such function as the probable duration of life, the probability of death in any year being as great as in any other. It confessedly errs greatly at the beginning and end of life, and is only a very rough approximation to the truth for the middle period of life.

Specific Intensity is a term employed by Mr. Neison (*Contributions to Vital Statistics*, 3rd edition, page 7) to represent the number living at any age divided by the number dying at that age. Thus, out of 100,000 males born, 76,504 survive at the age of 40 years, and lose during the year 927 of their number. The specific intensity at that age is therefore $\frac{76504}{927}=82{\cdot}508$. Both male and female life attain their highest specific intensity at the age of 14 years by Mr. Neison's table.

Probabilities of Life.—It is sometimes desirable to ascertain not only the probable duration of life, but also the probability of dying within a given period, or of a given disease. We now discuss, therefore, the methods of ascertaining the probabilities in these cases.

In mathematical language, the words *chance* and *probability* are used as synonymous; but in common language the first word is used when the expectation that an event will happen is small, and the second when it is large. In what follows, an elementary knowledge of the Theory of Probability, which is given in standard works on Algebra, is assumed.

If the number of possible events $=a+b$, of which a are favourable and b unfavourable, and if $p=$ the probability of a favourable event happening and q = the probability of an unfavourable event happening, then, on the supposition that one of these events happens, $p=\frac{a}{a+b}$; $q=\frac{b}{a+b}$; where $p+q=1$, or certainty.

Thus, if we wish to find the probability of a man aged 30 living till he is 50, and also the probability that he will die before that age, we consult the Life Table for males. From this we find that the number living (out of a million males born) at 30 is 630,038; at 50 is 476,980. Therefore the probability of a man aged 30 living to $50=\frac{476980}{630038}$.

And as $630038-476980=153058$ = the number dying during the period; therefore $\frac{153058}{630038}$, or $1-\frac{476980}{630038}$ = probability of dying between 30 and 50.

If there be several independent events, the probabilities of the happening of which are respectively p_1, p_2, p_3, etc., then the probability that all the events will happen is $p_1 \times p_2 \times p_3 \times$ etc.; that all will fail $(1-p_1)$ $(1-p_2)$ $(1-p_3)$ etc.; that at least one event will happen, $1-(1-p_1)$ $(1-p_2)$ $(1-p_3)$ etc.; and that exactly one will happen and all the rest fail, $p_1(1-p_2)$ $(1-p_3)$ etc. $+p_2(1-p_1)$ $(1-p_3)$ etc. $+p_3(1-p_1)$ $(1-p_2)$ etc. + etc.

Thus, if $p=\frac{a}{a+b}$ and $p_1=\frac{c}{c+d}$, then the probability that both will happen is $\frac{a}{a+b}\times\frac{c}{c+d}$, and the probability that neither will happen is this amount subtracted from unity.

Thus, the probability that a married couple—the husband's age being 40, and that of the wife 35—will both live 15 years, is obtained as follows:—

By Dr. Ogle's Life Table, out of 1,000,000 of each sex at birth, there are—

Of males at 40 years old, 563,077; at 55 years old, 424,577.
Of females „ 35 „ 628,842; „ 50 „ 520,901.

The probability of both these persons surviving 15 years from their present age $=\frac{424677}{563077}\times\frac{520901}{628842}$, which product gives the required result.

Next, as to the *probability of dying from a given disease.*

In Dr. Farr's 35th Supplement to the Report of the Registrar-General is given a table derived from the English Life Table No. 3, in which the deaths from 25 more important diseases are separately stated for different groups of ages. In such a Life-Table population the disturbing effect of an excess of young persons in the population on the mortality from various diseases is eliminated. Thus, if it is required to find the probability that a live-born child will die of scarlet fever during the first five years of life,—

By table 7, p. xciv., of the above report, of 1,000,000 children born, 17,959 die of scarlet fever between birth and their sixth birthday. Therefore probability of dying of scarlet fever between 0 and $5=\frac{17959}{1000000}=\frac{1}{55}$ nearly.

Similarly, to find the probability of a person dying at any age of scarlet fever. Total number of deaths from scarlet fever to a million deaths is 30,021. Therefore probability of dying from scarlet fever at some age $=\frac{30021}{1000000}=\frac{1}{33}$.

Similarly, the probability that a person will die of phthisis $=\frac{114417}{1000000}=\frac{1}{8}$ nearly.

To find the probability that a person aged 25 will die of phthisis.

Number out of a million at birth living at age 25 = 634045.

Number dying subsequently of phthisis = 81424.

The probability of dying of phthisis $=\frac{81424}{634045}=\cdot 12842=\frac{1}{8}$ nearly.

There is, therefore nearly 1 chance to 7 that the person

will die of phthisis, and 7 to 1 that he will die of some other disease.

The probability that a live-born child will die of any of the 25 diseases given in Dr. Farr's table is as follows:—

Smallpox	·006521	Diseases of Heart & Dropsy	·076660
Measles	·012865	Diseases of Lungs	·149585
Scarlet Fever	·030021	Diseases of Lungs and Phthisis	·264002
Diphtheria	·004945		
Whooping Cough	·015161	Diseases of Stomach and Liver	·052497
Typhus	·038107		
Diarrhœa and Dysentery	·034366	Diseases of Kidneys	·014910
Cholera	·006155	Diseases of Generative Organs	·003062
Other Zymotic Diseases (Order I.)	·027478	Diseases of Joints	·003395
Cancer	·021311	Diseases of Skin	·002512
Scrofula and Tabes	·014106	Childbirth and Metria	·006921
Phthisis	·114417	Suicide	·003479
Hydrocephalus	·011252	Other Violent Deaths	·030052
Diseases of Brain	·121859	Other Causes	·198363

CHAPTER XVI.

THE DECLINE IN THE ENGLISH DEATH-RATE AND ITS CAUSES.

Ages at which Decline in Death-Rate has Occurred.—Effect on Mean Duration of Life.—Life-Table Comparison the only Accurate Method.—Effect of Extinction of any Disease on Mean Duration of Life.—Causes of Greater Mortality at Higher Ages.—Expectation of Life for each Year of Age.—Balance of Loss and Gain between Old and New English Life-Tables.—Causes of Increased and Decreased Mortality.

WE have in a former chapter dwelt on the fall in the general death-rate, following on the passing of the Public Health Act (page 125 *et seq.*). The decline in the English death-rate has also been ably treated in the Registrar-General's Report for 1879, and in Dr. Ogle's Supplement to the 45th Annual Report for 1871–80; in a paper by Mr. N. A. Humphreys, read before the Statistical Society, April, 1883, on "The Recent Decline in the English Death-Rate, and its Effect on the Duration of Life"; and in a paper read before the same Society, March, 1884, by Dr. G. B. Longstaff, on "The Recent Decline in the English Death-Rate considered in connection with the Causes of Death."

Before discussing the subject in detail, the following table may with advantage be studied. From this, it will be evident that there has been a remarkable decline in the general death-rate. During the years 1841–70, the death-rate of males averaged 23·3 per 1,000, and during 1881–85 only 20·4, equal to a decline of 12·44 per cent. The death-rate of females fell from 21·4 in 1841–70 to 18·2 in 1881–85, equal to a decline of

14·95 per cent. Two other facts come out prominently in this table, viz., the marked decrease of the death-rate among the young, and especially in childhood, and the somewhat increased death-rate among adults.

Mean Annual Death-Rate per 1,000 *in England and Wales at Twelve Groups of Ages, in Groups of Years.*

Ages.	Mean Annual Death-Rate of Males.				Mean Annual Death-Rate of Females.			
	1841–70	1871–5	1876–80	1881–85	1841–70	1871–75	1876–80	1881–85
All Ages.	23·3	23·3	22·2	20·4	21·4	20·7	19·5	18·2
0–5	72·5	70·0	67·2	59·6	62·7	60·0	57·0	50·5
5–10	8·6	7·2	6·4	5·8	8·4	6·6	6·0	5·6
10–15	4·8	4·0	3·5	3·2	5·0	4·0	3·6	3·3
15–20	6·7	5·7	5·0	4·6	7·3	6·0	5·1	4·7
20–25	8·9	8·1	6·8	6·0	8·6	7·5	6·3	5·9
25–35	9·8	10·1	8·7	8·2	10·1	9·2	7·9	7·9
35–45	13·0	14·3	13·5	12·7	12·4	12·0	11·2	10·9
45–55	18·5	20·1	19·0	19·4	15·7	15·8	14·9	15·2
55–65	32·0	34·7	34·6	33·6	27·8	28·8	28·9	27·8
65–75	66·7	69·4	67·6	68·8	59·7	61·0	60·2	59·5
75–85	147·4	148·0	146·7	144·6	135·1	134·3	132·3	129·4
85 and upwards.	311·6	315·0	304·1	296·4	288·8	285·9	274·0	267·8

The influence on the mean duration of life of this change in the mortality at different ages requires careful consideration.

In order to this, however, it is necessary to take two periods for which Life Tables have been constructed. The first period taken is 1838–54, on the basis of which Dr. Farr's English Life Table No. 3 was constructed. For the second period we might select 1876–80, for which Mr. Humphreys constructed a special Life Table, but we prefer to take Dr. Ogle's table for 1871–80, as it is founded on more extensive and consequently more trustworthy data, though Dr. Ogle's results are, on the whole, identical with those of Mr. Humphreys. The following table gives a comparison between the death-rate at different ages periods at these two periods.

Mean Annual Mortality of Males and Females in 1838–54 *and in* 1871–80, *showing the Increase or Decrease per cent.*

Groups of Ages.	Males.			Females.		
	Mean Annual Death-Rate per 1,000 Living.		Increase or Decrease per cent.	Mean Annual Death-Rate per 1,000 Living.		Increase or Decrease per cent.
	1838–54	1871–80		1838–54	1871–80	
All Ages.	23·28	22·61	−2·88	21·65	20·00	−7·62
0–5	72·50	68·14	−6·01	62·28	58·10	−6·71
5–10	9·20	6·67	−27·50	9·11	6·20	−31·94
10–15	5·17	3·69	−28·62	5·38	3·70	−29·40
15–20	7·11	5·23	−26·44	8·53	5·43	−36·34
20–25	9·46	7·32	−22·62	9·05	6·78	−25·08
25–35	9·99	9·30	−6·91	10·55	8·58	−18·67
35–45	12·83	13·74	+7·09	12·70	11·58	−8·82
45–55	18·51	20·05	+8·37	15·87	15·59	+1·76
55–65	31·83	34·76	+9·26	28·16	28·54	+1·35
65–75	66·89	69·57	+4·01	59·99	60·82	+1·39
75–85	147·58	150·80	+2·18	134·37	135·40	+0·22
85 and upwards.	308·21	327·40	+5·91	288·16	296·40	+2·86

It will be seen that, as regards the general mortality, there was a reduction of 2·88 per cent. for males, and of 7·62 per cent. for females. The mortality of males was reduced in 1871–80 up to the 25–35 age-period, the greatest reduction being between 10 and 25 years of age, reaching as high as 28·62 per cent. between 10 and 15. The mortality of females was reduced up to the 35–45 age-period, and not only reduced during a greater portion of life, but to a greater extent, than the male mortality amounting to as much as 36·34 per cent. in the 15–20 age-period. The increase in female mortality at the higher ages was not so considerable as that of males, so that on the whole females have gained much more than males by the decreased mortality.

Before entering on a discussion of the subject whether the changes in the death-rates have been advantageous to the community, it may be well to discuss two preliminary questions; viz., the effect of the extinction of any single disease on the duration of life, and the causes of the greater mortality in adult life.

Effect of Extinction of any Disease on the Duration of Life.—In a Life-Table population, the mean after-lifetime, or mean duration of life at birth, is found by dividing the sum of the number of years the entire population lives by the number of persons. The extinction of any disease might theoretically produce two results on the mean duration of life. Either (1) the proportion of deaths from other causes would remain as before; or (2) if one disease be annihilated (as, for instance, smallpox), other diseases (as scarlet fever and measles) would become more fatal, thus counterbalancing to a greater or lesser extent the gain.

If all the deaths now caused by violence were to cease, the persons thus saved would doubtless share the rate of mortality of the whole community. If, again, the causes of death annihilated are those peculiar to children in the first year of life (as convulsions, premature birth, etc.), then, supposing that 100,000 lives are saved in this way out of a million born, and that these 100,000 children live an average lifetime, the expectation of life by the English Life Table No. 3 will be raised by one-tenth; *i.e.*, instead of 40·9 years, will become 45 years. It may be assumed as probable, however, that the lowered mortality in childhood saves some lives which carry through their later years comparatively unsound constitutions, and thus the *rate* of mortality at the higher ages is increased. The *actual* mortality must necessarily be increased at the higher ages; for all men must die at some time, and the larger the number escaping the dangers of childhood, the more numerous will be the victims to mortality in adult life. But the larger proportion living (on the supposition just made) to adult life need not theoretically have a higher death-*rate*, and the explanation of this higher death-rate will require consideration a little later.

If we imagine the extinction of such a disease as cancer, which is chiefly fatal after the age of 45, it is evident that no addition will be made to the years lived by those under 45 in a Life-Table population. Up to this age, no appreciable difference will be produced; but there being one less prospective enemy to encounter in the later years of life, the expectation of life at birth will be somewhat extended. The extinction of cancer, however, would not have so great an effect on the mean expectation of life as the extinction of zymotic diseases, which are especially fatal in the early years of life, or of phthisis, which particularly affects middle life. This for two reasons: first, because the absolute number of deaths from cancer is fewer than the number from phthisis or zymotic diseases; and secondly, because the population decreases with the advance of age, and consequently the number affected by the extinction of a given disease also decreases. Dr. Farr has worked out by the Life-Table method the effect of excluding from the general mortality deaths from zymotic diseases, from phthisis, and from cancer separately, and the following table gives his results for males :—

Four Life Tables for Males (calculated from the facts recorded in 1860–71), *showing the effect of the Exclusion of Deaths from* (1) *Zymotic Diseases,* (2) *Phthisis, and* (3) *Cancer, on the probabilities of living from age to age.*

Age.	Living at Each Age.				Dying in Each Interval of Age.			
	To Die of all Diseases.	Order I. of Zymotic Diseases Excluded.	Phthisis Excluded.	Cancer Excluded.	Of all Diseases.	Order I. of Zymotic Diseases Excluded.	Phthisis Excluded.	Cancer Excluded.
0	510,622	510,622	510,622	510,622	142,805	99,272	140,977	142.787
5	367,817	411,350	369,645	367,835	14,688	7,479	13,997	14,670
10	353,129	403,871	355,648	353,165	7,788	5,934	6,798	7,772
15	345,341	397,937	348,850	345,393	10,474	9,533	6,857	10,442
20	334,867	388,404	341,993	334,951	13,854	13,566	7,725	13,325
25	321,013	374,838	334,268	321,126	30,258	31,164	18,868	30,094
35	290,755	343,674	315,400	291,032	36,617	39,107	28,010	36,142
45	254,138	304,567	287,390	254,890	44,313	48,846	40,798	43,327
55	209,825	255,721	246,592	211,563	58,981	67,133	63,367	57,618
65	150,844	188,588	183,225	153,945	73,435	87,442	87,279	73,444
75	77,409	101,146	95,946	80,501	59,583	76,002	73,695	61,531
85	17,826	25,144	22,251	18,970	17,037	23,948	21,305	18,147
95	789	1,196	946	823	780	1,187	937	814
105	9	9	9	9	9	9	9	9

It will be seen from this table that if Order I. of zymotic diseases (miasmatic diseases) be excluded from the mortality, of 510,622 boys born, 411,350 will live to the age of 5, 343,674 to the age of 35, and similarly for the other diseases. The mean expectation of life by the exclusion of miasmatic diseases would be raised from 39·68 to 46·77 years; by the exclusion of phthisis, would be raised to 42·96 years; by the exclusion of cancer, to 39·88 years. Now the total number of deaths in the foregoing Life-Table population for males from miasmatic diseases is 89,192; from phthisis, 56,856; and from cancer, 6,794. Thus the greatest proportional effect on the mean duration of life will be produced by the elimination of zymotic diseases, which are most fatal in the early years of life: the next greatest by the exclusion of phthisis, a disease especially fatal in middle life; and the least by the exclusion of cancer, a disease setting in after the age for phthisis.

The Greater Mortality of Adult Life in Recent Years.—We have already alluded to one possible cause of this. The recent decline in the death-rate has been almost exclusively in the early years of life. This has probably resulted in the survival of a number of weakly children, who carry with them through life an enfeebled constitution, and thus tend to lower the average healthiness of the adult classes and increase their average death-rate. But the same causes which have lowered the mortality at the earlier ages *have also improved the average health of those who survive.* The wounded as well as the killed are fewer in number. Which of these two counteracting influences is the most potent,—the survival of a larger number of weakly ones, or the improved health of the general mass of the community,—must be regarded as still a matter of speculation.

Dr. Ogle mentions two other possible causes of this increased adult mortality. The increasing severity of competition among adults, resulting in greater wear and tear of life, tends to shorten life; and the ever-increasing proportion of the population which flocks to share in city life has a most important influence in the same direction. In regard to the latter cause, it should be noted that although the urban rate of mortality has diminished more rapidly and greatly than the rural mortality (page 136), "urbanization" is still an important cause of high mortality.

Gain or Loss from Changes in Incidence of Mortality.—We may now return to the question, whether this alteration in the rate of mortality at different age-groups has been on the whole advantageous to the community. The death-rate has increased for males over 35, and for females over 45, and it would therefore appear at first sight that for a large portion of what may be called the useful or non-dependent lifetime there is a distinct loss. But such a view of the matter loses sight of the important fact that a *larger proportion of those born survive to the non-dependent or useful ages.* This is brought out by the Life Table; and the only non-fallacious method of studying this question is by means of a Life Table founded on the number living and the number dying at each age.

Dr. Ogle's Life Table (Supplement to 45th Annual Report of Registrar-General, pp. vii. and viii.) contrasts the number surviving at each age with the corresponding number by Dr. Farr's Life Tables, and we may compare the results in the two cases. Taking first the **male Life Table**, by the old table one-half out of a million males born would be dead before the end of the 45th year; by the new table half would not have died until after the end of the 47th year. Taking each age in succession, it will be seen that the survivors at the end of each year, by the new table, exceed the survivors of the same age by the old table at every age up to the 67th year, and that the surviving males at the end of the 67th year from birth are, by the new table, 267,829, while the survivors by the old table are 267,160. After that date, the survivors at the end of each subsequent year are more numerous by the old than by the new table. Thus a male child, subject to the rates that prevailed in 1871–80 has a better chance of living 67 years than one subject to the rates that prevailed in 1838–54, but a smaller chance of living more than 67 years. It will be plain from what has been said that the fact that the death-rate of males after 35–45 has increased does not imply that the number of males surviving from a given number at starting will be less after that age. The real fact, as pointed out by Dr. Ogle, is that the survivors at the end of the 45th year are so much more numerous than they were under the rate of mortality prevailing in 1838–54, that "they can support the higher mortality of after years for a considerable period and yet retain their numerical superiority."

Next let us compare the expectation of life by the old and new tables. In the following table the expectation of males and females is given for each year of life according to Dr. Ogle's Life Table, and in the next column is given the increase or decrease of this expectation of life, as compared with the old Life Table (No. 3 of Dr. Farr). By subtracting the amounts marked +, and adding the amounts marked – to the expectation of life by the new table, the corresponding expectation by the old table is obtained. The expectation of life of an average male at birth by the new table is 41·35, by the old table 39·91 years, showing an average gain of nearly a year and a half for each male. The after-lifetime of males is longer by the new table at each year till the 19th. At the close of the 19th year it is 40·17 years by each table. After this age the individual male lives a shorter time than he did formerly; but *the aggregate life is considerably greater*, owing to the much greater number who survive to live these shorter lives.

If we next take the **female Life Table**, by the old table half out of a million women born die before the end of the 47th year from birth; whereas by the new table half live until the end of the 52nd year. The number of survivors by the new table is larger at every age up to the end of the 92nd year of life, and this spite of the fact that the female death-rate has increased after the 45–55 age-period. Thus a female born in 1871–80 had a slightly better chance of living to be 92 than one born in 1838–54, but a slightly less chance of living longer than that. In regard to expectation of life, there is at birth an average gain of 2·77 years for each female. From the preceding table it will be seen that the after-lifetime is longer by the new table to the completion of the 45th year, when it is 24·06 years by both tables; after this age the after-lifetime is shorter by the new table than by the old.

Age.	Males.		Females.	
	Expectation of Life or Mean After Lifetime.	Increase or Decrease since 1838-54.	Expectation of Life or Mean After Lifetime.	Increase or Decrease since 1838-54.
0	41·35	+1·44	44·62	+2·77
1	48·05	+1·40	50·14	+2 83
2	50·14	+1·31	52·22	+2·82
3	50·86	+1·25	52·99	+2·79
4	51·01	+1·20	53·20	+2·77
5	50·87	+1·16	53·08	+2·75
6	50·38	+0·99	52·56	+2·56
7	49·77	+0·85	51·94	+2·41
8	49·10	+0·73	51·26	+2·28
9	48·37	+0·63	50·53	+2·18
10	47·60	+0·55	49·76	+2·09
11	46·79	+0·48	48·96	+2·01
12	45·96	+0·42	48·13	+1·93
13	45·11	+0·35	47·30	+1·86
14	44·26	+0·29	46·47	+1·81
15	43·41	+0·23	45 63	+1·73
16	42·58	+0·18	44·81	+1·67
17	41·76	+0·12	44·00	+1·60
18	40·96	+0·06	43·21	+1·54
19	40·17	0·00	42·43	+1·46
20	39·40	−0·08	41·66	+1·37
21	38.64	−0·16	40·92	+1·29
22	37·89	−0·24	40·18	+1·25
23	37·15	−0·31	39·44	+1·11
24	36·41	−0·38	38·71	+1·03
25	35·68	−0·44	37·98	+0·94
26	34·96	−0·48	37·26	+0·87
27	34·24	−0·53	36·54	+0·79
28	33·52	−0·56	35·83	+0·73
29	32·81	−0·62	35·11	+0·65
30	32·10	−0·66	34·41	+0·60
31	31·40	−0·69	33·70	+0·53
32	30·71	−0·71	33·00	+0·47
33	30·01	−0·73	32·30	+0·42
34	29·33	−0·74	31·60	+0·37
35	28·64	−0·76	30·90	+0·31
36	27·96	−0·77	30·21	+0·27
37	27·29	−0·77	29·52	+0·23
38	26·62	−0·77	28·83	+0·19
39	25·96	−0·76	28·15	+0·16
40	25·30	−0.76	27·46	+0·12
41	24·65	−0·74	26·78	+0·09
42	24·00	−0·73	26·10	+0·07
43	23·35	−0·72	25·42	+0·04
44	22·71	−0·70	24·74	+0·02
45	22·07	−0·69	24·06	0·00
46	21·44	−0·67	23·38	−0·02
47	20·80	−0·66	22·71	−0·03
48	20·18	−0·64	22·03	−0·05
49	19·55	−0·62	21·36	−0·06
50	18·93	−0·61	20·68	−0·07

Age.	Males.		Females.	
	Expectation of Life or Mean After Lifetime.	Increase or Decrease since 1838-54.	Expectation of Life or Mean After Lifetime.	Increase or Decrease since 1838-54.
51	18·31	−0·59	20·01	−0·08
52	17·71	−0·57	19·34	−0·08
53	17·12	−0·55	18·66	−0 09
54	16·53	−0·53	17·98	−0·10
55	15·95	−0·50	17·33	−0·10
56	15·37	−0·49	16·69	−0·10
57	14·80	−0·46	16·06	−0·11
58	14·24	−0·44	15·45	−0·10
59	13·68	−0·42	14·84	−0·10
60	13·14	−0 39	14·24	−0·10
61	12·60	−0·36	13·65	−0·10
62	12·07	−0·34	13·08	−0·09
63	11·56	−0·31	12 51	−0·09
64	11·05	−0 29	11·96	−0·09
65	10·55	−0·27	11·42	−0·07
66	10·07	−0·25	10·90	−0·08
67	9·60	−0·23	10·39	−0·08
68	9·14	−0·22	9·89	−0·08
69	8·70	−0·20	9·41	−0·07
70	8·27	−0·18	8·95	−0·07
71	7·85	−0·18	8·50	−0·07
72	7·45	−0·17	8·07	−0·06
73	7·07	−0·15	7·65	−0·06
74	6 70	−0 15	7·25	−0·06
75	6·34	−0·15	6·87	−0·06
76	6·00	−0·15	6·51	−0·05
77	5·68	−0·14	6·16	−0·05
78	5·37	−0·14	5·82	−0·06
79	5·07	−0·14	5·50	−0·06
80	4·79	−0·14	5·20	−0·06
81	4·51	−0·15	4·90	−0·08
82	4·26	−0·15	4·63	−0 08
83	4·01	−0·16	4·37	−0·08
84	3·58	−0·37	4·12	−0·09
85	3·56	−0·17	3·88	−0·10
86	3·36	−0·17	3·66	−0·10
87	3·17	−0·17	3·46	−0·10
88	2·99	−0·17	3·26	−0·10
89	2·82	−0·18	3·08	−0·10
90	2·66	−0·18	2·90	−0·11
91	2·51	−0·18	2·74	−0·11
92	2·37	−0·18	2·58	−0·12
93	2·24	−0·17	2·44	−0·11
94	2·12	−0·17	2·30	−0·12
95	2·01	−0·16	2·17	−0·12
96	1·90	−0·16	2·11	−0·06
97	1·81	−0·14	2·03	−0·03
98	1·72	−0·13	1·83	−0·13
99	1·65	−0·11	1·73	−0·13
100	1·61	−0·07	1·62	−0·14

Balance of Loss and Gain.—In a Life Table the number of years lived by a million males starting at birth is equal to the sum of the number living at each age beyond 0, until each individual member of the million has died. Now if in the old and new Life Tables a summation is thus made of the years lived in each respectively, it is found that according to the new table a million males would live 1,439,139 more years than would be the case according to the old table. Similarly, a million females would live 2,777,584 additional years. The distribution in time of the years thus gained is given by Dr. Ogle as follows:—

Additional Years Lived by a Million Males and a Million Females.

Age-Periods.	Males.	Females.
0–15	255,340	288,226
15–25	281,872	339,933
25–35	344,906	453,221
35–45	310,746	499,471
45–55	211,040	474,009
55–65	86,920	385,257
65–75	–10,464	239,617
75–85	–27,770	89,568
85 and upwards	–13,451	8,282
Total years gained	1,439,139	2,777,584

The preceding table completely disposes of the mistaken notion that because the death-rates have fallen only in the earlier age-periods the aggregate gain to the community is confined to the dependent or unproductive years of life. If 25–65 years of age be taken as the most valuable part of life, a calculation founded on the above table shows that of the aggregate years saved, 66 per cent. in the case of males, and 65 per cent. in the case of females, are lived between 25 and 65 (Ogle). Dr. Ogle gives a further calculation, based on the preceding data, showing the *actual annual gain*, owing to the lower death-rate in 1871–80. The mean annual number of births in England and Wales in 1871–80 was 858,878, of which 437,492 were male and 421,386 female. If these children be traced throughout life, the changes in the death-rates occurring in 1871–80, as compared with 1838–54, would result in an addition of 1,800,047 years of life shared among them; and since this number of births occurs annually, it may be reasonably inferred that there is an annual addition of nearly two million years of life to the community, the greater share in which must be ascribed to sanitary measures.

Distribution of Decreased Mortality according to Cause.—In the following table the mortality of 1871–80, from certain defined causes, is contrasted with that of the preceding decennium. The contrast would have been more striking if we had taken the years of the present decennium instead of

Annual Deaths per Million Living in two Decennia.

Cause of Death.	1861-70	1871-80	Annual Increase or Decrease in 1871-80.
Small Pox	163	236	+73
Measles	440	378	−62
Scarlet Fever	972	716	−256
Diphtheria	185	121	−64
Whooping Cough	527	512	−15
Fever	885	484	−401
Diarrhœal Diseases	1,076	935	−141
Cancer	387	473	+86
Phthisis	2,475	2,116	−359
Hydrocephalus	347	317	−30
Other Tubercular Diseases	437	445	+8
Diseases of the Nervous System	2,785	2,770	−15
,, ,, Circulatory System and Dropsy	1,349	1,477	+128
,, ,, Respiratory System	3,364	3,760	+396
,, ,, Digestive System	981	978	−3
,, ,, Urinary System	298	392	+94
Puerperal Fever, Childbirth	165	167	+2
Violence	765	733	−32
All other and Unstated Causes	4,815	4,262	−553
All Causes	22,416	21,272	
Balance of Decrease			1,144

T

1871–80, and the materials for such a comparison will be found on page 172. The rate of mortality for 1861–70, from different causes, may be regarded as very similar to that for 1838–54, and the following table may therefore, with approximate accuracy, be regarded as a comparison applying to the same facts as the old and new English Life Tables.

It will be seen that in the aggregate zymotic diseases show a considerable decrease, fever showing a very remarkable decline. Among the other named diseases, the most striking features are the great decrease in phthisis, and the increase under the head of respiratory, circulatory, and urinary diseases. The mortality from these various causes has been already discussed at page 217.

CHAPTER XVII.

STATISTICS OF SICKNESS.

Incapacitating Sickness.—Time Lost by Sickness per Annum.—Statistics of Friendly Societies.—Number Constantly Sick per Cent.—Economical Aspect of Sickness.—Expectation of Sickness.—Duration of Attacks of Sickness.

WE have in Chapter iii. discussed the subject of registration of sickness, and at page 40 have given the rates of sickness for towns in which compulsory notification of infectious diseases is enforced, as compiled by Dr. Tatham.

The materials are lacking for a complete study of the amount of illness in the community, in the absence of any complete system of registration of disease; and estimates of the amount of illness have been based mainly on the records of sick-clubs and benefit societies, and the official returns of the Army, Navy, and Police.

No distinct line of demarcation exists between health and sickness, and the two are connected by a series of intermediate states. Only sickness which is sufficiently severe to involve confinement to bed or house, or to incapacitate for labour, is in practice capable of being registered; and even in regard to this disabling sickness our information is very partial.

The following table, from the article by Dr. Farr in McCulloch's "Account of the British Empire" (1854), shows the time lost by sickness and by accidental injury among the labourers in Portsmouth and Woolwich dockyards:—

	Mean Number of Workmen.	Days Lost by Sickness.	Days Lost by Accidents.	Constantly Sick per Cent.	Constantly Suffering from Accidents per Cent.	Constantly Ill from both Causes per Cent.
Portsmouth.	5,939	27,410	15,590	1·26	0·73	1·99
Woolwich .	2,243	10,593	8,594	1·29	1·05	2·34

The statistics collected in these dockyards (1830-32) gave the following results, as summarized by Dr. Farr: In each year one man in six was seriously hurt; two in five fell ill; and each man, on an average, had every two years an attack of illness, either spontaneous or caused by external injury. As seen in the previous table, at least 2 per cent. of the labourers were constantly disabled, two-thirds of this number being dependent on spontaneous disease.

Days of Sickness per Annum.—In his address at the inauguration of the International Health Exhibition, 1884, Sir James Paget gave the following table, prepared for him by the Actuary to the Registry of Friendly Societies:—

Ages.	Population of England and Wales, Census 1881.		Weeks' Sickness per Annum, according to the Experience of the Manchester Unity.		Average Sickness per Individual per Annum (in Weeks).	
	Males.	Females.	Males.	Females.	Males.	Females.
15 to 20	1,268,269	1,278,963	844,428	851,701	·666	·666
20 to 25	1,112,354	1,215,872	820,183	896,685	·737	·737
25 to 45	3,239,432	3,494,782	3,224,134	3,476,146	·995	·995
45 to 65	1,755,819	1,951,713	4,803,760	5,368,229	2 736	2·751
All Ages, from 15 to 65 .	7,375,874	7,941,330	9,692,505	10,592,761	1·314	1·334

This table is founded on the experience of the largest and most important of the Friendly Societies—the Manchester Unity of Oddfellows; and gives a calculation of the average annual rate of sickness of each person enumerated at the census of 1881 as living between the ages of 15 and 65, on the assumption that the rates of sickness of the whole population during the working years of life (15 to 65) would not be very different from the sickness rates of this Society.

The table shows that among males during the working years of life the average annual time of sickness is 1·314 weeks, or a fraction more than 9 days in each year; in females a fraction more. The total annual loss of work through sickness among males is 9,692,505 weeks; among females, 10,592,761 weeks, or about twenty millions of weeks altogether. This estimate is founded on the experience of nearly 400,000 members of the Manchester Unity; and as these may be regarded as in some measure insured lives, and as belonging to the more frugal portion of the working classes, their experience may be regarded as approximately correct for the whole community. Very few of the insane, or imbecile and idiotic, are included in the Society of the Manchester Unity of Oddfellows, and it is to be remembered that there are about 70,000 of these in our population doing no work, and losing not less than 3½ millions of weeks' work in the year (Paget).

From the same source, we have a calculation of the number of days for which each member of these Societies, when "off work" on account of sickness, receives a money allowance founded on the experience of *all* the registered Friendly Societies. The average number of days' sickness per member per annum is very nearly 1½ weeks, according to Mr. Sutton, the actuary to the Registry of Friendly Societies, a calculation which nearly agrees with the results of Mr. Neison's earlier elaborate researches. For further tabular statements, see Appendix, II. and III., pp. 316, 317.

Number Constantly Sick.—The following table shows the proportion of disabling sickness according to the returns of various Friendly Societies, and the corresponding figures relating to the East India Company's labourers (McCulloch's Account, 1854).

Average Number Constantly Sick to 100 *Living at each Age.*

Ages.	Friendly Societies.				East India Company's Labourers.
	Scotland (Highland Society).	England (Ansell).	Scotland (Neison).	England (Neison).	
20–30	1·14	1·54	1·65	1·69	1·62
30–40	1·32	1·83	1·63	1·91	2·06
40–50	1·97	2·56	2·44	2·89	2·69
50-60	3·00	4·32	5·17	5·21	6·58

Thus, by the experience of the English Friendly Societies, according to Neison's tables, between the ages of 20 and 30, out of 100 units of lifetime (days, weeks, or years), 1·69 were lost by disabling sickness, and from 50 to 60 the loss was 5·21 per cent.

The amount of sickness experienced in the thirty years of life, from 20 to 50, is, by the Highland Society's returns, 22 weeks; by Ansell's returns, 31 weeks; Neison's, 33 weeks; and by the same returns, from 30 to 60 years of age, it is 34 weeks, 45 weeks, and 52 weeks respectively.

Dr. Farr, in his Supplement to the 35th Annual Report of the Registrar-General, estimates that in England to one annual death in a body of men, two are on an average constantly suffering from sickness of some severity. Thus there are on an average two years of severe sickness to one death. According to some Friendly Societies the constantly sick to one annual death are 2·8. These exact relations between sickness and mortality are probably not preserved at the extremes of life, but they may be accepted as an approximation to the truth. On the basis of these data, it may be calculated that, inasmuch as in 1887 there were in the United Kingdom 693,843 deaths, there were 1,387,686 constant sufferers from severe sickness, and nearly two million sufferers from such illness as would require medical relief, or throw the members of Friendly Societies on their funds. Now the estimated population of the United Kingdom was 37,075,963, and this must be reduced by two millions to obtain the number of those in the enjoyment of health and capacity for work.

The amount of sickness represented by these figures implies an immense pecuniary loss to the State, which is hardly realized. When we remember that a large proportion of this sickness is preventible, the necessity of increased efforts to improve the unfavourable conditions under which a large proportion of the population lives becomes emphasized.

The unnecessary loss of life and resources begins with infancy, and holds throughout the more useful working periods of life. Even Malthus, with his advocacy of restraint of population, was impressed with the wastefulness of a high infantile mortality. He says: "A large birth-rate, together with a large infantile death-rate, is most wasteful to a State, as a large part of its produce would be distributed without return to children who would never reach manhood. A young person saved from death is more likely to contribute to the creation of resources than another birth. It is a great loss of labour and food to begin over again."

A still greater economical loss to the community is caused by the preventible sickness and mortality from 15 to 45 years of age. Thus, by Dr. Farr's English Life Table, of a million children born, 72,397 die between the ages of 15 and 45 as the result of phthisis, and 24,805 as the result of zymotic diseases. Dr. Ransome calculates that at least 40,000 to 50,000 lives are lost every year from alcoholic indulgence. Each of these annual deaths implies the constant sickness of two persons during the year. Premature death is an evil and a loss to the State, but sickness is from an economical aspect a still greater evil; for sickness adds an additional burden, while death can but remove the bread-winner.

The pecuniary value of each member of the community varies with age; but if we take the money value of each person aged 15 to 45 as £200 (see page 14), the pecuniary loss from phthisis alone at these ages, according to Farr's Life Table, is for every million children born 72,397 × 200 = £14,479,400.

During 1887 phthisis caused, between 15 and 45 years of age, 29,771 deaths (a smaller number than would have occurred according to Farr's Life Table, owing to the fact that the mortality from phthisis is on the decline). These deaths imply a loss of £5,954,200.

Expectation of Sickness.—The following table gives the expectation of sickness at different ages according to Dr. Southey, and may be compared with the somewhat similar figures given by Mr. Sutton on page 276:—

Expectation of Sickness.

Age in Years.	Days Ill Annually.
20	4
20–30	5–6
45	7
50	9–10
55	12–13
60	16
65	31
70	74

Duration of Sickness.—The following table, prepared by Mr. G. P. Neison from the returns of the Scotch Friendly Societies (page 164, 3rd edition, *Contributions to Vital Statistics*), gives the average duration in weeks of total sickness at different groups of ages :—

Average Duration in Weeks of Attacks of Sickness.

Age.	Total Number of Attacks, including those ending in Recovery and those ending in Death.	Total Amount of Sickness, including that ending in Recovery and that ending in Death.	Average Duration of each Attack of Total Sickness, including that ending in Recovery and that ending in Death.
10–15	12	39·428	3·286
15–20	117	749·571	6·407
20–25	637	2830·285	4·443
25–30	985	5483·000	5·566
30–35	1074	5014 143	4·668
35–40	872	4524·714	5·188
40–45	758	4158·714	5·486
45–50	519	3445·714	6·639
50–55	537	6634·285	12·354
55–60	491	7171·571	14·608
60–65	350	9102·286	26·004
65–70	135	5934·714	43·960
70–75	116	8867·999	76·448
75–80	29	4588·857	158·236
80–85	19	4027·000	211·947
85–90	...	...	...
90–95	1	353·000	353·000
All Ages 10–95	6652	72925·281	10·959

It will be seen that the duration of sickness, whether ending in death or not, is less protracted at the younger and middle periods of life than at the more advanced.

In another table, of which the following is a condensation, Mr. Neison distinguishes between the sickness preceding death and that followed by recovery. The previous table represents the average duration of sickness in 6,652 attacks of sickness, of which 5,640 recovered and 1,012 attacks (among 437 persons) ended in death, either during the course of that single illness or during the twelve years over which the observations extended.

Average Duration in Weeks of each Attack of Sickness.

Age.	Ending in Recovery.	Not ending in Death, but among those afterwards Dying during the Twelve Years of Observation.	Immediately Preceding Death.	Among those Dying, including the Attacks immediately preceding Death and others.
Col.	1.	2.	3.	4.
10–35	4·372	7·872	14·907	11·031
35–50	5·131	7·228	12·006	9·276
50–60	11·717	8·711	34·851	18·789
60 & upwds.	44·794	7·236	122·708	60·990
Total	8 636	7·888	45·173	23·932

Thus, of the attacks of sickness ending in recovery, the average duration is 8·636 weeks, being only 4·372 weeks under the age of 35, and increasing rapidly with age. It would appear from column 2 that up to the age of 50 the duration of each attack of sickness ending in recovery is greater among those who die within the period of observation (twelve years) to which the above table relates, *i.e.*, among those whose ultimate death is comparatively near, than among those who survive beyond the period of observation.

The sickness statistics of the Army and Navy are the most trustworthy and complete at our command. They will be considered, along with the other vital statistics of the two services, in the next chapter. Enthetic disease (mainly syphilis and gonorrhœa) is not recognised by Friendly Societies as constituting a claim to sick allowance; but in the Army and Navy we shall find that it greatly swells the rate of sickness.

See also Appendix, II. and III. (pp. 316, 317).

CHAPTER XVIII.

ARMY AND NAVY STATISTICS.

Average Strength of Army.—Rates of Mortality and Sickness in Army.—Average Sick-Time.—Causes of Sickness.—Ratio of Invaliding.—Duration of Service and Age of Invalided.—Average Strength of Navy.—Rates of Sickness, Invaliding and Mortality.—Causes of Sickness in Navy.

ARMY STATISTICS.—The following statistics concerning the Army are derived from the Army Medical Department Report for the year 1886.

The average annual strength of the troops serving at home and abroad during this year was 188,739 warrant officers, non-commissioned officers and men (exclusive of certain regiments in Malta, West Indies, Ceylon, and Hong-Kong, which were recruited locally). The admissions into hospital in this force

White Troops.	Average Strength.	Admitted into Hospital.	Died.	Sent Home as Invalids.	Discharged as Invalids.	Constantly non-effective from Sickness.
Troops at Home and Abroad	**188,739**	**204,792**	**2,189**	**2,610**	**2,828**	**10,743·52**
United Kingdom	92,601	78,089	632	—	1,667	4360·31
Gibraltar	4,307	3,634	41	116	30	211·38
Malta	4,736	3,435	34	77	59	220·82
Cyprus	636	682	7	7	—	32·32
Egypt	11,062	14,070	408	928	270	820·54
Canada	1,283	751	3	23	20	38·77
Bermuda	1,227	781	15	20	20	42·30
West Indies	1,020	1,192	15	14	12	56·19
Cape of Good Hope and St. Helena	3,971	3,211	17	78	51	194·95
Mauritius	414	597	9	16	6	31·38
Ceylon	949	1,079	10	14	10	58·55
China and Straits Settlements	2,269	2,665	26	22	20	112·12
India	61,757	91,630	958	1,300	663	4563·89
On board Ship	2,507	2,976	14	—	—	—

were 204,792, and the deaths 2,189. These give a rate for admissions into hospital of 1,085·1, and for deaths 11·48 per 1,000 of the average annual strength.

In the preceding table the average strength of the troops in different parts of the British Empire is stated, with the statistics relating to mortality, invaliding, and non-effectiveness from sickness.

Rates of Mortality and Sickness in the Army per 1,000 *of Strength.*

	Rates per 1,000 of Strength.					Average Annual Sickness to each Soldier.	Average Duration of each Case of Sickness.
	Admitted into Hospital.	Died.	Sent Home as Invalids.	Discharged as Invalids.	Constantly non-effective from Sickness.		
						Days.	Days.
Troops at Home and Abroad 1876–85	1072·2	11·70	38·50	21·39	52·36	19·11	17·74
Troops at Home and Abroad 1886	1085·1	11·48	27 88	15·03	57·69	21 06	19·43
	*	†	‡	§	‖	‖	‖
Troops in United Kingdom 1876–85	847·0	6·93	—	25 07	44·56	16·26	19·20
Troops in United Kingdom 1886	843·3	6·68	—	17·64	47·08	17·18	20·38
Foreign Troops 1886—							
Gibraltar	843·7	9·51	26·93	6·96	49·07	17·91	21·23
Malta	725·2	7·17	16·25	12·45	46·62	17 02	23·46
Cyprus	107·23	11·00	11·00	—	50·81	18·55	17·30
Egypt	127·19	36·88	83·89	24·40	74·17	27·07	21·28
Canada	585·3	2·34	17·93	15·59	30 22	11·03	18·84
Bermuda	636 5	12·22	16·29	16·29	34·47	12·58	19·77
West Indies	1168·6	14·70	13·73	11·76	55·09	20·11	17·21
Cape of Good Hope and St. Helena	808·6	4·28	18·38	12·84	49·09	17·91	22 16
Mauritius	1442·0	21·73	38·64	14·49	75·79	27·66	19·18
Ceylon	1136·9	10·53	14·75	10·53	61 68	22·52	19·81
China and Straits Settlements	1174 5	11·45	9·69	8·81	49·41	18·03	15·35
India	1483·7	15·51	21·05	10·73	73·90	26.97	18·18
On Board Ship	1187·1	5·58	—	—	—	—	—

* Calculated on strength, excluding men detached (1,900).

† Calculated on strength, including men detached.

‡ Calculated on strength, excluding United Kingdom and troops on board ship.

§ Calculated on strength, including men detached, and excluding troops on board ship.

‖ Calculations exclude men detached and troops on board ship.

In the foregoing table the rates per 1,000 of average strength are shown for 1886, as compared with the average of the preceding ten years.

The statistics for the United Kingdom show that the average strength of the Army at home during 1886 was 92,601. The average number of daily sick was 4,360·31, the average sick-time to each soldier 17·18 days per annum, and the average duration of each case of sickness 20·38 days. The average sick-time to each soldier was shorter than the corresponding period in the preceding year by half a day, but the average duration of each case of sickness was longer by about one-fifth of a day. The following table shows the chief causes of the 78,089 admissions into hospital in the United Kingdom during 1886, also the number constantly sick and the number dying during the year in proportion to 1,000 of the troops.

Disease or Injury.	Admissions into Hospital during 1886.	Ratio per 1,000.	
		Constantly Sick.	Deaths.
Smallpox	11	·01	—
Other Eruptive Fevers	598	·30	·02
Enteric Fever	145	·25	·46
Other Continued Fevers	842	·37	·09
Dysentery	87	·10	·06
Malarial Fevers	562	·23	—
Syphilis { Primary	8.236	7·75	—
Syphilis { Secondary	3,097	2·59	·05
Gonorrhœa	10,632	7·05	—
Alcoholism	308	·08	·07
Rheumatism	3,709	2 53	·04
Tubercular Diseases	362	·61	1·17
Diseases of the Nervous System	924	·94	·48
„ „ Eye	1,281	·80	—
„ „ Circulatory System	835	·82	·53
„ „ Respiratory „	7,323	3 88	1·83
„ „ Digestive „	9,233	3·10	·49
„ „ Generative „	4,814	2·97	·04
„ „ Skin „	8,450	3·26	—
Other Diseases	7,662	5.33	·51
Injuries	8,978	4·11	·84
General Total.	73,089	47·08	6·68

The total number discharged the service by invaliding during 1886 was 1,667, being in the ratio of 17·64 per 1,000 of the strength, which is lower than the corresponding rate in the previous year by 3·97, and than the decennial average rate by 25·07 per 1,000. The most frequent causes of invaliding were diseases of the circulatory system, 298 men, or 3·15 per 1,000 being discharged on this account. Next in order come diseases of the nervous system with a rate for invaliding of 2·77 per 1,000 (1·31 per 1,000 for mental disease); and tubercular diseases with a rate of 1·60 per 1,000.

The number invalided during each period of service in the Army is shown in the following table. The ratios of invaliding

Duration of Service in Army.	Number Invalided.	Strength of Army of this Term of Service.	Ratio of Number Invalided to 1,000 of Strength.
First Year	383	30,236	12·66
0–5 years	1,041	69,430	14·99
5–10 ,,	279	13,935	20·02
10–15 ,,	81	5,658	14·31
15–20 ,,	199	6,616	30·07
Over 20 ,,	67	2,404	27·87
All Periods	1,667	98,043	17·64

in the later periods are higher than in earlier periods, on account of the number of older soldiers discharged out of a comparatively small strength.

Age at Time of Invaliding.	Number Invalided.	Strength of Army of this Age.	Ratio of Number Invalided to 1,000 of Strength.
Under 20 years of age	256	27,901	9·17
20–25 ,, ,,	665	40,754	16·32
25–30 ,, ,,	366	14,892	24·58
30–35 ,, ,,	122	6,626	18·41
35–40 ,, ,,	179	5,955	30·06
Over 40 ,, ,,	79	1,915	41·25
All Ages	1,667	98,043	17·64

The number invalided at different ages is shown in the preceding table.

The strength of the Army in the United Kingdom, as given in this table, does not correspond with the strength as given in the table on page 283 (92,601), the discrepancy being due in part to the inclusion of detached men, and in part to other causes not explained by the Director-General in his report.

The table on page 288 shows the admissions, deaths, number invalided, and number constantly sick, in each portion of the home force, with the ratios per 1,000 of the strength, and the corresponding ratios for the average of the previous ten years.

The average strength of officers during 1886 was 3,644, the number of attacks of sickness 1,177, and the number of deaths 23. The ratio of prevalence of sickness was therefore 323·0, and of mortality 6·31 per 1,000. The corresponding death-rate for the whole Army in the United Kingdom was 6·68 per 1,000.

The rate of mortality of the troops serving in the United Kingdom, like that of the general population of England and Wales, varies greatly at different groups of ages. In the following table the death-rate per 1,000 for the home Army at different groups of ages is stated. We have found it impracticable to compare these with the death-rates at different groups of ages for the civil population, because the groups of ages do not correspond, and because the totals on which the death-

		Annual Death-Rate per 1,000 Living at the following Ages.					
		Under 20.	20–25.	25–30.	30–35.	35–40.	40 & Upwards.
Troops on Home Service	Mean of 1876–85	3·10	4·78	6·19	9·79	14·97	22·86
	1886	3·87	5·29	7·08	10·46	12·79	25·11

rates at different ages in the army have been calculated, are not given. The fallacy involved in compounding and combin-

Vital Statistics of the Army in Great Britain.

Arms of the Service.	Average Strength.	Admitted into Hospital.	Died.	Discharged as Invalids.	Average Number Constantly Sick.	Annual Ratio per 1,000 of Strength.				Average of 10 Years, 1876–85.			
						Admitted.	Died.	Invalided.	Constantly Sick.	Admitted.	Died.	Invalided.	Con-stantly Sick.
Household Cavalry .	1,275	805	6	32	44·40	631·4	4·71	25·10	34·82	658·6	3·73	23·46	34·50 *
Cavalry .	10,119	9,398	50	230	520·88	928·7	4·94	22·73	51·48	929·7	5·61	30·55	49·66 *
Royal Artillery .	15,532	12,126	137	352	734·56	780·7	8·82	22·66	47·29	768·0	7·58	25·18	42·80 *
Royal Engineers .	3,174	1,909	16	43	121·57	601·4	5·04	13·55	38·30	599·0 ‡	7·65	18·17	31·86 †
Foot Guards	5,535	5,500	29	139	344·91	993·7	5·24	25·11	62·31	979·0	7·27	24·00	53·46 *
Infantry .	37,677	34,295	220	611	1936·91	910·2	5·84	16·22	51·41	878·9	6·42	26·32	48·06 *
Regimental Depôts .	13,592	10,172	122	196	421·86	748·4	8·98	14·42	31·04	858·8	10·77	28·92	38·41 *
Garrison Staff and Departments .	5,697	3,884	52	64	235·22	681.8	9·13	11·23	41·29	595·5 ‡	7·94	15·73	37·73 †

* For eight years only. † For seven years only. ‡ For nine years only.

ing death-rates, instead of dealing with the totals on which these rates are calculated, will be dealt with in the next chapter (p. 309).

Navy Statistics.—The following particulars are obtained from the Statistical Report of the Health of the Navy for 1887. The total force in the service afloat was 48,410 officers and men. This includes men on short leave of absence, and the sick under treatment in hospital. These were included in the estimate for the first time, thus increasing the force by about 3 per cent. as compared with that of former years. If computed as in former years, the force would have been 46,958. The effect of this difference on the death and other rates may be seen in the following tabular statement:—

Total Force Calculated According to	Ratio per 1,000 of the Naval Force.		
	Of Cases of Sickness and Injury.	Of Invalidings.	Of Deaths.
New Method (48,410) . .	1018·81	50·15	8·32
Old Method (46,958) . .	1050·32	51·09	8·58

The distribution of the force according to age was as follows:—

Age.	Number of Troops.	Percentage of Total Troops.	Death-Rate per 1,000 in 1887.
15–25	26,470	54·67	7·4
25–35	15,740	32·51	8·19
35–45	5,110	10·55	12·13
Over 45	1,090	2·25	14·67
All Ages	48,410	100·	8·32

The rates of mortality, of invaliding, and of cases of sickness per 1,000 of the force at each of these groups of ages, in different stations of the service at home and abroad is shown in the following table:—

Stations.	Ratio per 1,000 of Force of Cases placed on the Sick-List.		Ratio per 1,000 of Force Invalided.		Ratio of Deaths per 1,000 of Force.	
	For the Year 1887.	Average Ratio for Ten Years.	For the Year 1887.	Average Ratio for Ten Years.	For the Year 1887.	Average Ratio for Ten Years.
Home	812·4	872·38	24·76	31·7	5·73	6·39
Mediterranean	1105·63	1343·89	51·76	56·44	9·68	8·07
North America and West Indies	1100·37	1261·44	34·07	35·47	6·29	6·19
South-East Coast of America	779·24	1285·42	11·32	28·92	5·66	6·67
Pacific	1080·64	1195·17	20·64	28·34	4·51	5·
West Coast of Africa and Cape of Good Hope	1217·44	1256·34	41·86	41·29	6·97	11·66
East Indies	1773·18	1602·21	71·36	60·52	9·09	13·23
China	1287·36	1530·68	27·19	29·17	6·04	8·87
Australia	1480·	1230·63	18·06	24·	9·67	6·9
Irregular	1119·26	1306·73	18·09	33·05	22·56	22·53
Total Force	1018·81	1125·27	30·15	36·6	8·32	9·19

The total number of cases of disease and injury entered on the sick-list was 49,321, which is in the ratio of 1018·8 per 1,000. On the average 2,133 men were sick daily, which is in the ratio of 44·06 per 1,000. The total number of days of sickness, on board ship and in hospital, in the total force, was 778,556, giving an average annual loss of service from sickness and injury of 16·08 days for each person, showing a decrease of 0·83 in comparison with the average of the last ten years.

The total number of persons invalided was 1,460, or 30·15 per 1,000. Of this total, 928 persons were finally invalided out of the service, being in the ratio of 19·16 per 1,000 of the whole force, or 63·56 per cent. of the number invalided. Of the total number invalided, 1,350 were invalided for disease, and 110 for injury.

The number of deaths during 1887 was 403, which gives a ratio of 8·32 per 1,000, showing a decrease of 0·87 on the average of the last ten years. The geographical distribution of sickness and mortality is clearly shown in the preceding table, which will repay study. Of the total deaths, 237 were due to disease, and 166 to injury; the death-rate from disease being 4·89, and from injury 3·42 per 1,000.

The chief causes of illness and death in the entire Navy are shown in the following table:—

Disease or Injury.	Number of Cases during 1887.	Rates per 1,000 of Strength.	
		Cases.	Deaths.
Smallpox	1	·02	—
Other Eruptive Fevers	199	4·11	·06
Enteric Fever	138	2·85	·76
Other Continued Fevers	1,611	33·27	·02
Dysentery	108	2·23	·10
Malarial Fevers	1,651	34·1	·30
Syphilis { Primary	2,924	60·4	—
Syphilis { Secondary	934	19·29	·02
Gonorrhœa	3,598	74·32	—
Effects of Climate	159	3·28	—
Alcoholism	64	1·32	·04
Rheumatism	2,188	45·19	·04
Tubercular Diseases	9	·18	·12
Diseases of the Nervous System	793	16·37	·28
,, ,, Eye	528	10·9	·88
,, ,, Circulatory System	307	6·34	·24
,, ,, Respiratory ,,	4,140	85·51	1·79
,, ,, Digestive ,,	6,236	128·81	·39
,, ,, Urinary & Generative System	660	13·63	·35
,, ,, Connective Tissue and Skin	10,552	217·97	—
Other Diseases	1,929	—	—
Injuries	10,572	218·37	3·29
General Total	49,321	1018·81	8·32

CHAPTER XIX.

STATISTICAL FALLACIES.

Quetelet's Rules.—Fallacies already Exposed.—Classification of Fallacies.—Fallacies from Paucity of Data.—Poisson's Formula.—Fallacies owing to Inaccurate or Incomparable Data.—*Non Ceteris Paribus.*—Alleged Deterioration of Recruits.—Comparison of Deaths without Correction for Alteration of Population.—Fallacies concerning Averages.—Mean and Extreme Values.—Mean Strength.—Hospital Statistics.—Bed and Patient Death-Rate.

THE reservation of an entire chapter to the consideration of the fallacies into which those who employ figures frequently fall appears almost as absurd as it would be to devote a chapter at the end of a treatise on grammar to the consideration of grammatical errors. The study of the science of grammar involves the exposure of grammatical errors; and similarly, if we have been successful in our attempt to treat of the principles of Vital Statistics, the fallacies which we so frequently meet with in medical statistics may be considered already sufficiently exposed. But while this is logically correct, there is a practical convenience in presenting a concise summary of the more important statistical errors, and especially so as this will enable us to consider in detail several cases which have not arisen in the preceding chapters.

We may first of all cite Quetelet's four chief rules, which are worthy to be held in remembrance.

1. Never have preconceived ideas as to what the figures are to prove.

2. Never reject a number that seems contrary to what you might expect, merely because it departs a good deal from the apparent average.

3. Be careful to weigh and record *all* the possible causes of an event, and do not attribute to one what is really the result of the combination of several.

4. Never compare data which have nothing in common.

Were these rules constantly followed, the science of statistics would be much more respected than it is, and the value of its results would be greatly increased.

Errors already Exposed.—In the preceding chapters, numerous instances have arisen, illustrating various phases of statistical fallacies. Before considering other cases, it may be well to recapitulate those already mentioned.

Population forms an essential datum in the presentation of all Vital Statistics, and inaccurate estimates of population vitiate every subsequent calculation. Instances of such inaccurate estimates are given at p. 7. The errors arising in connection with the statement of age, infirmities, etc., are given at pp. 2, 3, and 103. The age and sex constitution of the population has a great influence on the marriage-rate (p. 43), on the birth-rate (p. 55), and on the death-rate (p. 90); and unless due allowance be made for variation in composition of the population as to age and sex, especially as to age, serious errors will arise.

A correct and complete registration of causes of death is another essential datum in the presentation of Vital Statistics, and the chief errors in this connection have been already discussed (p. 21).

The questions of increase of cancer (p. 208), and of decrease of phthisis (p. 212) involve serious statistical difficulties, which have been already considered. The fallaciousness of the assumption that a fixed ratio exists between sickness and mortality has been discussed (pp. 31, 177).

We have stated that the birth-rate, to be strictly accurate, should be calculated in terms of the number of women living at child-bearing years (p. 55), and that the number of illegitimate births should not be stated in proportion to the total births (p. 63).

The fallacies connected with death-rates for short periods

have been pointed out (p. 75), as also the effect of migration of population in disturbing the death-rate (p. 77), the effect of public institutions on the same (p. 81), and the fallacies as to the correct relationship of birth-rate to death-rate (p. 83). False methods of estimating the mortality at different ages have been exposed (p. 100). The sources of error in connection with occupational statistics are discussed at page 153, and, among other additional fallacies which have been considered, we may mention those in regard to smallpox (p. 191 *et seq.*), and in regard to the duration of life as evidenced by the mean age at death (p. 245).

Classification of Fallacies.—Without attempting a complete logical classification of fallacies, we may divide them into *fallacies of observation* and *fallacies of inference.* The errors which we shall consider will be found to come under one of these heads, in some cases illustrating them both, the data and the inferences from them being each inaccurate or incomplete, or both.

Errors from Paucity of Data.—The number of observations on which any deduction is founded should be considerable. The deduction is trustworthy in proportion as the observations are numerous, on the assumption that the latter are at the same time accurate and comparable. There is, unfortunately, nothing more common in medical literature than a crude generalization from insufficient data, especially as to the treatment of disease, ignoring the mathematical rule that the relative values of two or more series are as the square roots of the numbers of observations; so that by increasing the number of observations in any inquiry, the accuracy increases as the square root of the number. The results obtained, even from a large number of observations, are, however, only an approximation to the truth, although the limits of error are reduced with each increase in the number of observations.

The degree of approximation to the truth of a varying number of observations can be estimated by means of **Poisson's formula.** This formula can, however, only be trusted in the ideal case of games of chance, in other cases forming an inadequate test of accuracy.

Let μ = total number of cases recorded,
m = number in one group,
n = number in the other group,
so that $m+n=\mu$.

The proportion of each group to the whole will be respectively $\frac{m}{\mu}$ and $\frac{n}{\mu}$. These proportions will vary within certain limits in succeeding instances, and the extent of variation will be within the proportion represented by—

$$\frac{m}{\mu}+2\sqrt{\frac{2\cdot m\cdot n}{\mu^3}}$$

$$\text{and } \frac{n}{\mu}-2\sqrt{\frac{2m\cdot n}{\mu^3}}$$

It is evident that the larger the value of μ (the total number of observations) the less will be the value of $2\sqrt{\frac{2\cdot m\cdot n}{\mu^3}}$ and the less will be the limits of error in the simple proportion $\frac{m}{\mu}$.

Thus if out of ten cases of cholera seven recover, how near is this to the true average of recoveries? Here the probability of recovering is represented by $\frac{7}{10}$, of dying by $\frac{3}{10}$. The possible error is given by the second half of Poisson's formula. Thus—

$$2\sqrt{\frac{2\,m\cdot n}{\mu^3}}=2\times\sqrt{\frac{2\times7\times3}{10^3}}=2\sqrt{\frac{42}{1000}}=\cdot4098$$

Thus the possible error is as ·4098 to unity, or, in other words, the error is greater than the number of deaths. What will be the possible variation in 100,000 cases on this basis?

The average, as stated, is 70,000 recoveries out of 100,000 cases; the possible error is 40,980; therefore the number of recoveries may be either 29,020 or 110,980, a conclusion which is an obvious absurdity.

If, however, 100 cases be collected, out of which 70 recover, the proportion is the same; but by Poisson's formula the error is only ·13 to unity, and the range of recoveries out of 100,000 cases will lie between—

$$70{,}000 + 13{,}000 = 83{,}000$$
$$\text{and } 70{,}000 - 13{,}000 = 57{,}000$$

If 1,000 cases are taken, of which 700 recover, the error will be only ·04 to unity, and the range of recoveries in 100,000 cases will lie between—

$$70{,}000 + 4{,}000 = 74{,}000$$
$$\text{and } 70{,}000 - 4{,}000 = 66{,}000$$

The following table will show more clearly how, with an increasing number of facts, the limits of possible error (assuming the accuracy of the facts recorded) steadily decrease.

Total Number of Cases.	Number of Recoveries.	Possible Number Recovering out of 100,000 Cases according to Poisson's Formula.
10	7	29,020 *or* 110,980
100	70	57,000 ,, 70,000
1,000	700	64,000 ,, 74,000
10,000	7,000	69,700 ,, 71,300
100,000	70,000	69,600 ,, 70,400
1000,000	700,000	69,870 ,, 70,130

It is evident that a small number of observations is inadequate to establish a conclusion; but inasmuch as the degree of accuracy increases only in the ratio of the square root of the number of observations, the mere repetition of observations beyond a certain number (10,000 in the previous table) is proportionately of small value, and after a time becomes practically useless.

Errors from Inaccuracy or Incomparability of Data.—Inaccuracy or incompleteness of data necessarily leads to fallacious conclusions. Apart altogether from any intentional deception, the trustworthiness and ability of the observer or recorder of a given set of facts is an important element in estimating the reliability of deductions from them. It is necessary that the data should be collected on a uniform plan, and should be of a strictly comparable nature. Any neglect in stating a single cause of variation in some of the facts may vitiate the entire conclusion. Thus it is well known that cholera is much less fatal towards the end of an epidemic than at its commencement. If, therefore, in stating the percentage of recoveries, under a given method of treatment, no mention was made of the period of the epidemic when the cases came under treatment, a trustworthy conclusion would be impossible. The neglect of the precaution that the phenomena or *events dealt with shall be strictly comparable* has given rise to the most valid objections which have been urged against the use of the numerical method in medicine.

Dr. T. Graham Balfour, F.R.S., in his inaugural address as President of the Statistical Society (November, 1888), has given an interesting instance, arising from the alleged deterioration of recruits, of the fallacy due to overlooking the condition of "**other things being equal,**" which we shall now summarize.

It is stated, on the authority of the Director-General of the Medical Army Department, that in the years 1860–64 inclusive, no fewer than 32,324 examinations of recruits were made by army-surgeons; and that the rejections from all causes were 371·67 per 1,000. During 1882–86, 132,563 men offered themselves for enlistment, of whom 415·58 per 1,000 were rejected, showing a marked increase in the proportion of rejections. Sir Thomas Crawford can explain this increase in the rejections in one way only: "the masses, from whom the army recruits are chiefly taken, are of an inferior physique to what they were twenty-five years ago." Dr. Balfour, however, instituted independent inquiries, which threw grave doubt on this conclusion, and satisfied him that a large proportion, at least, of the striking excess of rejections at the later period was due, not to an increase in the disabilities among the recruits examined, but partly to improvements introduced into the returns in 1864, by which they were made much more complete, and partly to changes instituted in 1879 and 1880 in the system of examination. Prior to 1860 there was no return of recruits examined and rejected at out-stations, and the proportion of recruits rejected was in consequence considerably lower in the official figures than the facts warranted. From 1860-64, in addition to returns of staff-surgeons of the districts, returns were received from medical officers in charge of regiments and depôts, but a statement of the recruits examined and rejected by civilian practitioners was still lacking. In 1864 this last anomaly was removed, and thereafter it became possible to state accurately the total number examined as recruits and the proportion rejected on medical grounds.

Certain other alterations in regulations affect the comparability of later and earlier figures concerning recruits. In 1880 the responsibility as to deficient height, under-chest measurement, and apparently incorrectly stated age, was transferred from the recruiting officer to the medical officer, which would doubtless tend to increase the number of rejections.

This transference to the medical officer of a duty previously discharged by the recruiting officer evidently introduces a new element into the medical returns, which ought to be omitted in any comparison of the results of the examinations with those of previous periods. Similarly, on one or two other points, alterations of regulations affect the comparability of the results of different periods. If, in order to institute comparisons, the rejections from the causes concerning which the regulations have altered be omitted, the following results are obtained:—

Years.	Rejections per 1,000 Recruits.
1864–9	398·2
1870–74	314·6
1875–79	289 2
1880–85	299·5

Thus in the last period there was a reduction of one-fourth compared with the first period, and the proportion was almost identical with the average of the intervening ten years. It is evident, therefore, that the statistics relating to recruits for the army, when submitted to analysis, do not bear out the conclusion that the lower classes, from whom recruits are chiefly derived, are of an inferior physique now to what they were twenty-five years ago. On the other hand, it would be equally unfair to draw from these figures the deduction that the physique of the lower classes has improved. Owing to the varying regulations in force in the army, it is impossible to arrange the results in a form which complies with the condition of "other things being equal."

Dr. Balfour then considers the question of the data relating to height and chest measurement. There are serious difficulties in instituting comparisons between different periods, owing to the fact that the minimum height of recruits to be enlisted is frequently varied, in accordance with the larger or smaller number required to complete the Army establishment. By omitting, however, the entries of men of the lower heights, a comparison becomes possible as in the following table:—

Proportion of Recruits per 1,000 Examined at Various Heights above 5 ft. 6 in.

Periods.	5 ft. 6 in.	5 ft. 7 in.	5 ft. 8 in.	5 ft. 9 in.	5 ft. 10 in.	5 ft. 11 in.	6 ft. and upwards.
1864–68	383·2	278·0	168·7	90·4	44·0	21·3	14·4
1881–85	373·7	274·6	175·4	96·7	44·2	21·1	14·1

If this is a fair test, then there has been an improvement in the physique of the recruits during the later period.

We may give one more instance of the necessity for ascertaining any changes in the Army regulations before drawing conclusions from the results furnished by different periods.

In 1864, the proportion of recruits rejected because of marks of corporal punishment or the letters D and B C (deserter and bad character) was 3·61 per 1,000 inspected; in 1865–69 it averaged 2·28, declining steadily to 0·16 in 1880–85. This might at first sight be regarded as an indication of improved morals in the class of men presenting themselves for enlistment; but, on further examination, the explanation is found to lie in the facts that by the Mutiny Act of 1868 the infliction of corporal punishment was abolished, except on active service or on board a ship; and in 1871 the marking of deserters with the letter D and men discharged the service as bad characters with the letters B C was abolished.

Errors in Comparing Total Deaths in Successive Years.—It is inaccurate to compare the number of total deaths or the number of deaths from any one disease with the corresponding number in any previous year unless some allowance is made for increase of population. *Cæteris paribus*, a larger population would supply a greater number of deaths than a smaller one. We shall now demonstrate the method by which *the number of deaths in any year may be compared with the decennial average of the ten preceding years, corrected for increase of population during the period*, taking as an example the number of deaths from measles in England and Wales in 1887, and the average number in the decennium in 1877–86.

The number of deaths from measles in 1887 = 16,765.

The average annual number of deaths from measles in the ten years 1877–86 = 10,549.

What was this average corrected for increase of population, in order to allow accurate comparison with the figures for 1887?

Now, the population of England and Wales in 1887 = 28,247,151.

The mean population of 1877–86, obtained by summation of the populations in each year and division by ten = 26,256,699. The deaths from measles in the decennium 1877–86 must therefore be raised in the proportion of 26,256,699 to 28,247,151, in order to bring them into true comparison with those of 1887.

$$\text{But } \frac{28247151}{26256699} = 1{\cdot}075.$$

By multiplying 10,549 by 1·075 we obtain 11,340, which represents the average annual number of deaths from measles during the decennium 1877–86, corrected for increase of population.

This number, subtracted from 16,765, gives 5,425, which is the excess of deaths from measles in 1887 as compared with the mean of the previous decennium.

The following table, from the Registrar-General's Annual Summary for 1887, shows the amount of life saved and the amount lost during 1887, in London, compared with the mean annual mortality in the preceding decennium, the correction we have just described having been made.

Diminution or Excess of Deaths in London during 1887, *compared with Annual Deaths in* 1877–86, *Corrected for Increase of Population.*

Cause of Death.	Diminution in 1887.	Excess in 1887.
Smallpox	1,132	—
Measles	—	459
Scarlet Fever	518	—
Typhus	61	—
Whooping-cough	261	—
Diphtheria	—	180
Simple and Ill-defined Fever	86	—
Enteric Fever	314	—
Diarrhœal Diseases	—	478
Cancer	—	302
Phthisis and Tubercular Diseases	2,015	—
Premature Birth	—	197
Diseases of Nervous System	929	—
Diseases of Circulatory System	—	708
Diseases of Respiratory System (including Croup)	1,834	—
Diseases of Urinary System	—	192
Childbirth and Puerperal Fever	49	—
Accident	151	—
Murder, Manslaughter	5	—
Suicide	—	22
All other Causes	1,813	—
	9,198	2,538
Balance of Diminution and Excess	9,660	—

Errors in Regard to Averages.—The larger the basis of facts on which an average is founded the more reliable it is. Accidental causes may produce large variations in a small series of observations, which become corrected when the facts are multiplied. It is on this principle that, spite of the great annual fluctuations in the receipts and expenditure of Insurance Societies, the results become equalized for a series of years.

Dr. Guy gives the following instance of the value of increasing the number of facts on which an average is based, from an investigation into the average age at death of members of the peerage and baronetage:—

Number of Facts.	Average Age at Death.		
	Maximum.	Minimum.	Range.
25	69·40	50·64	18·76
50	66·44	55·20	11·24
100	63·70	56·85	6·85
200	62·38	57·61	4·77
400	61·10	58·24	2·86
800	60·84	59·97	1·17
1,600	60·25		

If we assume the true average duration of life of the members of the peerage and baronetage who have attained 21 years to extend to 60 years, then, omitting decimal points, the following table shows the errors in excess or defect:—

Number of Facts.	Errors in Excess or Defect.
25	9½
50	5½
100	3½
200	2½
400	1½
800	0½

It may happen, however, that the first 25 observations in a

table like the preceding would give as correct an average as 800 observations; and there is always a balance of probability in favour of the average of even a small number of facts approximating more closely to the true average than to the extremes. The extreme values, that is, the two ends of the scale, of which the average is the middle, should also be noted. As Dr. Guy puts it, "averages are numerical expressions of probabilities; extreme values are expressions of possibilities." The possible range of the average obtained from a stated number of observations can always be ascertained by means of Poisson's formula, thus indicating the possible amount of error.

Although, as already stated, the average of a small number of facts may give a near approximation to the truth, such an average must be regarded as requiring a confirmation which the average from a large number of facts does not require. It is important to note also that *the results obtained from an average can never be applied to a particular case.* An average is the mean result from a number of instances, all of which may be either above or below it, so that it does not necessarily express the exact truth in regard to any one of the cases on which the average is founded.

The fallacies connected with the application of the results of a large number of cases to an individual instance are well known to insurance offices, and have been alluded to in the chapter on Life Tables. General results from a large aggregation of facts may be safely applied to a similar aggregation of facts; but their application to single cases is full of dangers. Thus, the mean duration of life, according to a Life Table, expresses with almost mathematical certainty the average age at death of the members of a community *taken one with another*, but is not necessarily accurate when applied to a single individual. All that we can safely conclude is, that the excess of those who live longer will be counterbalanced by the deficiency of years of those who die at an earlier age than the average.

Extremes, being the expression of possibilities, require a larger number of individual facts than averages to render them trustworthy. Dr. Guy gives an interesting instance of neglect of this rule. M. Orfila stated that it was possible approximately to determine the stature of the skeleton and of the body by measuring one of the long bones. He did not test this, however, by taking extreme cases, but only by a rough average. It was subsequently found that out of seven ulnas, measuring in length 10 inches and 8 lines, one corresponded to a stature of 6 ft. $1\frac{1}{4}$ in., another to 5 ft. 5 in., implying a possible error of $8\frac{1}{4}$ inches.

In connection with Public Health, two fallacious uses of averages must be discussed, viz., the fallacy of average strength, and of bed-mortality in hospitals, which are closely connected.

Errors in Connection with Average Strength.—The sickness and mortality statistics in the Army and Navy are calculated on what is known as the *average strength* or *mean force*. It is not quite clear, from the annual report of the Army Medical Department, whether the mean force includes those on sick leave as well as detached men, but apparently these are included. As already explained (page 289), in the Navy the mean force has been recently made to include men on short terms of leave of absence and the sick under treatment in hospital—a change which has been found to increase the force by 3 per cent. According to Dr. Parkes, the average strength includes in the Army the number of men of each regiment present at each station on the muster days, divided by the number of muster days. It thus includes the sick men in hospital as well as the healthy men, and is consequently not a completely accurate basis on which to determine the amount of disease among the healthy men. When many changes of troops occur, it is often difficult to ascertain the mean strength, and erroneous calculations are consequently not uncommon. An example, quoted by Dr. Parkes from a paper by Dr. Balfour, may be cited, which is of special interest, inasmuch as it affords an instance in which an unhealthy station in India (Masulipatam) was credited with a more favourable rate of mortality than it was entitled to. The Madras Medical Board stated that the death-rate among all the European regiments in the Presidency, from January, 1813 to December, 1819, was 56·9 per 1,000; while that of the regiments at Masulipatam from 1813 to 1832 inclusive was 51·0 per 1,000; and they inferred that the rate of mortality having been somewhat lower than throughout the rest of the Presidency for such a period, there was reason for concluding that the station could not be considered under ordinary circumstances as unhealthy. In arriving at the preceding death-rate for Masulipatam, however, the fact had been lost sight of, that in several of the years between 1813 and 1832, the regiments were quartered at Masulipatam during part of the year only. Under such circumstances, in calculating the annual death-rate, only such a proportion of the mean annual strength should be taken as corresponded with the period during which the regiment was stationed there. If it was stationed there six months, the calculation should be based on half the strength; if nine months, on three-fourths of it, and so on.

When the necessary correction was made in the instance cited, the annual death-rate from 1813 to 1832 was found to average 63·94 per 1,000, instead of 51·00 as previously stated.

The error we have just described is similar to the assumption that, in a town with a population of 100,000 persons, and in which 3,000 deaths occurred during nine months, the annual death-rate is 30 per 1,000. The population should, of course, be reduced by one-fourth; and the annual death-rate, on the assumption that the same rate of mortality continues during the remaining three months of the year, is 40 per 1,000.

Fallacies of Hospital Statistics.—Much of the misapprehension which has arisen in medical literature concerning hospital mortality is owing to a lack of comprehension of the facts relating to average strength, which we have already adduced. The subject is discussed very lucidly in the 6th Report of Mr. (now Sir John) Simon to the Privy Council for 1863; and we cannot give a better view of it than by summarizing his argument, founded on an investigation made by Dr. Bristowe and Mr. Holmes into the sanitary conditions of, and results obtained in, various large hospitals.

To begin with, the word "healthy," as applied to a hospital, evidently cannot denote that its inmates shall be persons in health; nor that its inmates shall not have a high death-rate, for this is involved in the condition of the inmates. A "healthy" hospital is one "which does not *by any fault of its own* (whether *inherent fault*, as of site or construction; or *fault of keeping*, as dirtiness or overcrowding) aggravate ever so little the sickness, nor oppose ever so little the recovery of persons who are properly its inmates."

Death is unquestionably the most serious form in which lack of success in treatment is evidenced. It is essential, however, if hospital death-rates are to possess the slightest value, that they should be calculated on *given magnitudes of illness*. The comparison of the death-rate in a fever hospital with that in an orthopœdic hospital would obviously be absurd. Unless due regard be had, therefore, to the uncertain import of the word "patient," death-rates are worthless as evidence of success or failure in hospital treatment. It is notorious that hospitals, with regard to the quality and magnitude of the cases received in them for treatment, differ enormously from one another. Large urban hospitals receive patients at any time and of the gravest character, and "wage an ever-precarious contest against the least conquerable forms of disease;" while in many country hospitals admission is by subscriber's letter, there is a comparatively infrequent change of patients, and a minimum of severe or urgent cases. On the whole, it may be safely asserted that the hospitals with high death-rates have no reason to be ashamed, nor the hospitals with low death-rates to congratulate themselves.

The Registrar-General published in his 24th Annual Report some statistics of the different hospitals. The census on April 8th, 1861, showed how many special inmates were contained in each of the hospitals of England, while the death-returns of the year 1861 showed how many deaths occurred during the year in the same hospitals. From these materials a general death-rate per 100 occupied beds, which may be called a *bed death-rate*, was compiled. Such bed death-rates are most misleading. (*a*) In the first place, they were calculated on the hospital population of a single day—that of the census, which may have been much above or below the average,—and not on the average daily sick population. Dr. Buchanan showed that, accepting the number of inmates at the census day in 1861 as the basis of calculation, the bed death-rate of the London Fever Hospital in 1860 was nearly 30 per cent., in 1861 nearly 500 per cent., in 1862 nearly 2,000 per cent., and in 1863 nearly 1,400 per cent.

(*b*) Each bed in a hospital usually receives during the year a succession of patients. All that a bed death-rate means is that there occurs in every occupied bed in a hospital a certain number of deaths per annum. A bed death-rate of 100 per cent. per annum means that on an average one death occurs during the year in every occupied bed of the hospital.

Classification of Hospitals, according to their respective Sites and Sizes.	Actual or Average Number of Special Inmates in each Hospital on April 8th, 1861.	Estimated Bed Death-Rate for the year 1861, per 100 Occupied Beds.
24 London Hospitals	176	90·84
12 Hospitals in Large Towns	156	83·16
25 County and important Provincial Hospitals	90	39·41
HOSPITALS IN LARGE TOWNS.		
Bristol Royal Infirmary	224	56·25
Birmingham Queen's Hospital	135	58·52
Nottingham General Hospital	137	40·88
Liverpool Northern Hospital	101	128·71
Manchester Royal Infirmary	202	130·69
COUNTY AND IMPORTANT PROVINCIAL HOSPITALS.		
Brighton Sussex County Hospital	109	66·06
Headington, Oxon, Radcliffe Infirmary	133	24·81
Dorchester County Hospital	50	24·00
Devon and Exeter Hospital	181	25·41
Bath United Hospital	78	102·56
Leicester Infirmary	83	61·45
Swansea Infirmary	30	10·00

(*c*) These objections, however, are trifling when compared with the objections already stated against all general death-rates as measures of hospital healthiness. The preceding table, selected from the Registrar-General's report alluded to, shows the striking and suspicious disparity between the bed death-rates of different hospitals.

Thus the Nottingham Hospital has a bed death-rate under 41, while that of Manchester is over 130; at Swansea the death-rate is only 10, while at Bath it is 102, per 100 occupied beds.

These results are quite untrustworthy. Assuming that the mortality in urban hospitals is twice as great as in rural hospitals, then we might conclude any one of three things: "either (1) that the urban hospitals change their sick population twice as often as the rural hospitals, and that other conditions are equal; or (2) that in the urban hospitals the mean gravity of cases received for treatment is twice as great as in the rural hospitals, and that other conditions are equal; or (3) that in the urban hospitals the success of treatment of given magnitudes of disease is half as great as in the rural hospitals, and that other conditions are equal." In all probability the two first of these suppositions express the truth, though unfortunately Dr. Farr gave the authority of his name to the statement that general hospitals, by reason of "defects" which "render them ways of death to their inmates," do "not benefit mankind directly," but merely "as pathological observatories and medical schools;" and Miss Florence Nightingale, in her *Notes on Hospitals*, has accepted Dr. Farr's conclusions as valid. The real fact is that general death-rates are inapplicable as tests of true differences of hospital success, and ought never to have been employed for this purpose.

If general death-rates are employed at all in regard to hospitals, the true principle on which to calculate them is on the basis of the aggregate annual number of cases treated to a termination. This may be called the *patient death-rate*, as distinguished from the bed death-rate already described. There is no necessary connection between the range shown by bed death-rates in the preceding table and the range of patient death-rates in the same institutions. Whether the two ranges would correspond depends on whether *the average time of staying in hospital* is the same in the hospitals compared. But as a matter of fact the staying-time varies enormously in different hospitals, being usually shorter in larger hospitals, and shorter in hospitals where the proportion of acute cases is high. If the mean stay of patients in hospitals is known, *bed death-rates* may at once be converted into *patient death-rates* or *vice versâ.*

It follows from the preceding considerations that comparisons of hospital statistics, if they are to serve any useful purpose, must be in considerable detail. Not only should cases of like nature be compared, but, inasmuch as the mortality from many diseases varies with age, the age-constitution of the patients of the institutions under comparison should be noted. A typhus patient aged 55 is at least ten times as likely to die as a typhus patient aged 15. Similarly the success of the operation of lithotomy varies greatly at different ages.

The success of the major amputations again varies greatly according to the age of patients, and according to whether it is required as the result of injury or disease; and in regard to all statistics dealing with the results of treatment, it is desirable that the age and special circumstances of the individual facts should be fully stated.

Errors from the Composition of Ratios.—As a general rule, it is dangerous in dealing with death and other rates to combine or compound such rates. This error is so commonly fallen into that the following illustrations of the resulting mistakes cannot be considered superfluous:—

Thus the population of—

Battersea	was	125,091	and its death-rate	20·00
Putney	„	14,450	„ „ „	13·70
				33·70

Mean death-rate of the two = 16·85

This, however, is a most incorrect result. The true method is as follows :—

Battersea	population,	125,091 ;	deaths,	2,503
Putney	„	14,450 ;	„	199
		139,541		2,702

Therefore $\frac{2{,}702 \times 1{,}000}{139{,}541} = 19{\cdot}59$ is the true death-rate.

The true death-rate is thus seen to be much higher than that first obtained, owing to the fact that in the first calculation equal prominence is given to the healthiness of Putney and of Battersea, although Putney has only one-eighth of the entire population.

Another instructive and somewhat amusing instance is furnished by a correspondence in the *Times* during September, 1888. *X* wrote to the *Times* newspaper, and on the assumption that the death-rate in the British Army at home and abroad in 1885 was 11·12 per 1,000, and the death-rate of troops at home 6·68, argued gravely that the death-rate of troops abroad was therefore 4·44 per 1,000! *Y* wrote to correct this statement, and pointed out that if *X's* method were correct, then it would be equally true that if the death-rate of the English and Irish in the United Kingdom was 21 per 1,000 and that of the Irish 20 per 1,000, the mortality of the English was only 1 per 1,000; or if the death-rate of the Irish was over 21, then the English live for ever! *Y* then proceeded to maintain that the true mortality of the troops abroad was 15·56 per 1,000, without mentioning, as *Z* pointed out in a subsequent letter, that this was only correct when the troops at home and abroad were equal in number; on which *Y* replied that "rates per 1,000 are quite irrespective of numbers at home and abroad"—a conclusion which is true for rates regarded separately, but flagrantly false when applied to their composition. As this question of the composition of rates is one of considerable delicacy and importance, we shall here discuss it in detail.

The general problem to be considered is as follows:—Having given the death-rate of the component parts of a population, to find what is the death-rate for the whole.

Let $a+b$ = total number of population (or body of men, as in preceding example), where a and b represent the population of each part.

Also let x = death-rate per unit of the portion a,
and y = " " " " b,
Where x differs from y.

Then the number of deaths in $a = a \times x = ax$.
Also " " " " $b = b \times y = by$.

Therefore the total number of deaths in $(a+b) = ax + by$.

Hence, dividing by the total population, we obtain—

$\frac{ax+by}{a+b}$ = death-rate per unit for the whole.

If the two parts of the population are equal; *i.e.*, if $a=b$,

the death-rate for the whole $= \frac{ax+ay}{a+a} = \frac{a(x+y)}{2a} = \frac{x+y}{2}$,

which is the mean of the two rates x and y.

Hence, when the parts of which a population is composed are equal, the death-rate of the whole is the mean of the death-rates of the component parts.

But if a be twice as great as b; *i.e.*, if $a=2b$, then the formula $\frac{ax+by}{a+b}$ may be written $\frac{2bx+by}{2b+b} = \frac{b(2x+y)}{3b} = \frac{2x+y}{3}$ where evidently the death-rate for the whole is not the mean of the death-rates for the two parts.

From this it is evident that when the death-rates of the component parts of a population are given, the death-rate of the whole population will depend on the relative proportion existing between the component parts of the population; and any variation in these proportions will cause a corresponding variation in the total death-rate. In order, therefore, to ascertain the total death-rates from the death-rates of the parts, we must either know the actual population of each component part or their relative proportions.

Reverting once more to the formula already given,—viz., $\frac{ax+by}{a+b}$ = death-rate per unit of the population $(a+b)$,—it is evident that, where the total death-rate is given and the death-rate of one component part of the population, this same formula will enable us to find the death-rate of the remaining portion.

Thus, taking the example already quoted from the *Times* newspaper,—

The death-rate of the Army at home and abroad in 1885 (as given in the *Times* correspondence) = 11·12 per 1,000.

The death-rate of the Army at home = 6·68 per 1,000.

To find the death-rate of the Army abroad. From the Registrar-General's returns, we find the strength of the total Army in 1885 = 198,064; of the Army at home = 91,579; of the Army abroad = 105,748.

By the formula $\frac{ax+by}{a+b} = 11{\cdot}12 = \frac{91{,}579 \times 6{\cdot}68 + 105{,}748 \times y}{198{,}064}$,

From which we obtain the result that $y = 15$ nearly.

Similarly, having given the death-rate of the Army in the United Kingdom in 1887 to be 5·3 per 1,000, of the Army abroad 14·0, to find the death-rate of the total Army, the strength of the Army in the United Kingdom being 106,767 and of the Army abroad 102,807.

Death-rate of the whole Army

$$= \frac{ax+by}{a+b} = \frac{106{,}767 \times 5{\cdot}3 + 102{,}807 \times 14{\cdot}0}{106{,}767 + 102{,}807}.$$

$$= 9{\cdot}6.$$

The use of the death-rate per 1,000 instead of per unit in these calculations does not alter the result, as it affects both numerator and denominator equally.

Another example may be taken. Having given the population of the twenty-eight great towns (including London) as 9,398,273, and their death-rate per annum for the quarter ending 29th December, 1888, as 19·8 per 1,000, the population of London as 4,282,921, and its death-rate for the same period

18·9 per 1,000; to find the average death-rate for the other twenty-seven towns:—

Let z = total death-rate, then—

$$z=\frac{ax+by}{a+b}\text{; whence—}$$

$$ax+by=z(a+b),$$
$$by=z(a+b)-ax,$$
$$y=\frac{z(a+b)-ax}{b}.$$

$$\text{Therefore } y=\frac{19{\cdot}8(4{,}282{,}921+5{,}115{,}352)-18{\cdot}9\times 4{,}228{,}921}{5{,}115{,}352},$$
$$=\frac{105{,}138{,}598{\cdot}5}{5{,}115{,}352}=20{\cdot}5.$$

Fallacies arising from Stating Deaths in Proportion to Total Deaths.—These have already received consideration (pages 100, 111, 168). They present themselves under two heads. The deaths at one age are stated in proportion to the total deaths at all ages; or the deaths from one cause are stated in proportion to the total deaths from all causes. In both cases the same fallacy is involved. A relationship is attempted to be established *between two factors, both of which are variable* in value. An alteration in the total deaths on one hand, or in the deaths at one group of ages or from one cause on the other hand, might equally affect the proportion between the two, though the conclusions to be drawn in the two cases would by no means be necessarily identical.

We may add a further illustration of this fallacy, furnished by Mr. (now Sir Edwin) Chadwick's address to the Association of Sanitary Inspectors (August, 1888). He stated that among the gentry and professional persons the deaths of children under five years of age in Brighton formed 8·93 per cent. of the total deaths, while among the wage-earning classes they formed 45·44 per cent. From these facts he would infer that the conditions of life for persons of the upper classes are about five times $\left(\frac{45{\cdot}44}{8{\cdot}93}\right)$ as favourable among the well-to-do as among the poor.

Such a conclusion is by no means warranted by the facts. The numbers dying at different ages among two populations, *cæteris paribus*, vary with the number living at the same ages; so that with the greater population under five among the poor we should expect a higher percentage of deaths under five than among the well-to-do. Unless we know the relative population under five in each case, we are not justified in drawing any conclusion from the preceding figures. This instance may serve to emphasize what has been previously said as to the importance of stating the deaths at any group of ages in terms of the number living at the same group of ages, and not as a percentage of the total deaths.

The same authority, in the address alluded to, gives another comparison which is equally fallacious. For the wage classes in Brighton the mean age at death, he states, is 28·8 years, for the well-to-do 63 years. The facts that the poor have a much larger number of children than the rich, and that the rich are largely formed of persons who began life poor, but have gradually worked their way into comfortable circumstances, are entirely ignored in this erroneous method of comparison between the two classes.

These examples illustrate the importance of the method first formulated by Mr. Milne, that the total deaths must be stated in proportion to the total number living, and that this method must be applied at each group of ages. They also illustrate the importance of a complete and accurate knowledge of the age (and sex) constitution of the population, a subject which has been repeatedly dwelt on in this book, and which forms the keynote to the rational interpretation of Vital Statistics.

APPENDIX I.

Occupations of Males and Females in England and Wales at the Census in 1881, arranged in Groups.

Class	Persons engaged in—	Persons.	Males.	Females.
Class I. Professional.	Order 1.—The General or Local Government of the Country	104,592	97,222	7,370
	„ 2.—The Defence of the Country	124,580	124,530	50
	„ 3.—Professional Occupations, with their immediate Subordinates	417,903	229,203	188,700
Class II. Domestic.	„ 4.—Domestic Offices or Services	1,803,810	258,508	1,545,302
Class III. Commercial.	„ 5.—Commercial Occupations	316,865	308,391	8,474
	„ 6.—Conveyance of Men, Goods, and Messages	663,263	652,270	10,993
Class IV. Agricultural.	„ 7.—Agriculture	1,278,624	1,214,453	64,171
	„ 8.—Persons engaged about Animals	104,560	103,891	669
Class V. Industrial.	Persons working and dealing in—			
	„ 9.—Books, Prints, and Maps	105,042	89,130	15,912
	„ 10.—Machines and Implements	267,976	253,994	13,982
	„ 11.—Houses, Furniture, and Decorations	786,660	768,283	18,377
	„ 12.—Carriages and Harness	87,174	84,692	2,482
	„ 13.—Ships and Boats	54,080	53,967	113
	„ 14.—Chemicals and Compounds	43,015	38,597	4,418
	„ 15.—Tobacco and Pipes	22,175	12,862	9,313
	„ 16.—Food and Lodgings	629,371	503,344	126,027
	„ 17.—Textile Fabrics	1,053,648	463,024	590,624
	„ 18.—Dress	981,105	364,680	616,425
	„ 19.—Various Animal Substances	68,202	53,564	14,638
	„ 20.—Various Vegetable Substances	166,745	130,580	36,165
	„ 21.—Various Mineral Substances	1,277,592	1,212,491	65,101
	„ 22.—General or Unspecified Commodities	816,243	753,285	62,958
	„ 23.—Refuse Matters	14,339	12,685	1,654
Class VI. Indefinite and Non-Productive.	„ 24.—Persons without Specified Occupations	14,786,875	4,856,256	9,930,619
	Total	25,974,439	12,639,902	13,334,537

APPENDIX II.

Mortality and Sickness Experience of the Ancient Order of Foresters Friendly Society for the Five Years, 1871–75 *—Males (Neison).*

Ages.	Rural Districts.			Town Districts.		
	Number of Members Exposed to Risk.	Annual Death-Rate per 1,000.	Sickness (in Weeks) per Member per Annum.	Number of Members Exposed to Risk.	Annual Death-Rate per 1,000.	Sickness (in Weeks) per Member per Annum.
18–	5268	7·40	·926	2795	11·09	1·080
20–	73565·5	6·70	·799	52521	7·29	·833
25–	165420·5	7·07	·868	151314·5	7·88	·933
35–	105232·5	9·54	1·123	104893·5	11·30	1·227
45–	46675·5	14·44	1·584	45960·5	17·38	1·950
55–	17968·	28·16	3·222	16270·5	33·44	3·817
65–	6872·5	61·11	8·640	5215	66 92	10·565
75–	771·5	129·62	17·525	488	168·03	21·516
85–	14	214·28	22·551	30	66·67	16·800
95–	5	—	6·771	35	114·29	22·008
Totals	421793·	10·45	1·258	379523	12·04	1·410

Ages.	City Districts.			All Districts Combined.		
18–	2179	11·93	1·251	10242	9·37	1·037
20–	55525·0	8·52	·833	181612	7·43	·819
25–	201468·5	9·03	·927	518203·5	8·07	·910
35–	153200	13·56	1·342	363326	11 74	1·245
45–	63673·5	21·09	2·130	156309·5	18·02	1·914
55–	19781	36·65	4·127	54019·5	32·86	3·732
65–	4702·5	68·90	8·558	16790	65·10	9·215
75–	303	148·51	14·352	1562·5	145·28	18·157
85–	17	117·65	5·386	61	114·75	14·939
95–	—	—	—	40	100·00	20·103
Totals	703195·	13·65	1·404	1302166	12·14	1·358

APPENDIX III.

Sickness Statistics of the Hearts of Oak Benefit Society for 1886.

Ages.	Number of Members Sick out of each 100 Exposed to Risk.				Average Sickness per Member Exposed to Risk (Weeks).				Average Duration of Sickness per Member Sick (Weeks).			
	Full Pay.			Half Pay.	Full Pay.			Half Pay.	Full Pay.			Half Pay.
	Total Country Districts.	Metropolitan Districts.	All Districts.	All Districts.	Total Country Districts.	Metropolitan Districts.	All Districts.	All Districts.	Total Country Districts.	Metropolitan Districts.	All Districts.	All Districts.
15–20	15·01	13·29	14·22	—	·51	·46	·49	—	3·41	3·45	3·43	—
20–25	21·87	16·07	19·22	·32	·81	·60	·70	·03	3·70	3·72	3·71	8·79
25–30	21·66	17·90	19·92	·47	·86	·63	·75	·05	3·95	3·50	3·76	10·53
30–35	23·53	20·58	22·03	·69	1·02	·84	·93	·07	4·33	4·09	4·22	10·80
35–40	24·14	21·65	22·66	1·06	1·14	1·03	1·07	·11	4·70	4·75	4·74	10·58
40–45	25·65	24·13	24·71	1·39	1·33	1·19	1·24	·16	5·17	4·93	5·02	11·34
45–50	29·09	26·29	27·47	1·58	1·53	1·54	1·53	·18	5·25	5·84	5·58	11·11
50–55	31·81	30·41	31·12	3·04	2·11	1·91	2·01	·32	6·62	6·29	6·46	10·65
55–60	32·99	36·22	34·53	3·80	2·33	2·56	2·44	·43	7·07	7·05	7·07	11·40
60–65	37·57	38·82	38·16	6·94	3·18	3·23	3·21	·95	8·47	8·34	8·41	13·69
65–70	34·75	34·56	34·68	6·28	2·92	3·89	3·31	·68	8·39	11·24	9·54	10·86
70–75	29·85	41·67	35·97	10·07	4·19	4·51	4·36	·80	14·03	10 83	12·12	7·96
75–80	—	33·33	14·29	—	—	1·27	·55	—	—	3·80	3·80	—
All Ages	24·12	21·59	22·77	1·01	1·12	1·01	1·06	·11	4·65	4·65	4·65	10·96

INDEX.

Butler & Tanner. The Selwood Printing Works, Frome, and London.

For Product Safety Concerns and Information please contact our EU
representative GPSR@taylorandfrancis.com
Taylor & Francis Verlag GmbH, Kaufingerstraße 24, 80331 München, Germany

www.ingramcontent.com/pod-product-compliance
Lightning Source LLC
LaVergne TN
LVHW011110300926
849160LV00008B/334

9781138906587